BIG FAT LIES SKINNY WOMEN TELL

Find out What it Really Takes to

Have the Body of your Dreams

By Camille Hugh

Also by Camille Hugh

The Thigh Gap Hack

Bye-Bye Thunder Thighs

How to Lose Water Weight

The Easy Diet

The Skinny Girl Bible

Your FREE Gift

As a thank you gift for purchasing *"Big Fat Lies Skinny Women Tell"*, I would like to offer you FREE access to my newsletter.

When you sign up, you will receive regular fitness and nutrition tips and tricks from me, as well as videos and articles with up to date information on the latest products, reviews, accessories and more that I only think is worthy of being shared.

All of this will go straight to your inbox, so you never miss a thing!

To find out more information and sign up, visit www.thighgaphack.com

Note to Readers

The content of this book, by its very nature, is general, whereas each reader's situation is unique. Therefore, the purpose is to provide general information rather than to address individual situations, which books by their very nature cannot do.

This book proposes a program of diet and exercise based on the opinions and ideas of the author. It is intended to provide helpful and informative material on the subject addressed in the publication and is sold with the understanding that the author and publisher are not engaged in rendering medical, health, psychological, or any other kind of personal professional services or therapy in the book.

The reader should consult his or her qualified medical, health, psychological, or other competent professional before starting this or any other fitness program, particularly if you suffer from any medical condition or have any symptom that may require treatment.

As with any diet or exercise program, if at any time you experience any discomfort, stop immediately and consult your physician.

The author and publisher specifically disclaim all responsibility for any liability, loss, or risk, personal or otherwise, which is incurred as a consequence, directly or indirectly, of the use and application of any of the contents of this book.

Published in the United States by The Feminine Contour, LLC

www.thighgaphack.com

TABLE OF CONTENTS

Introduction

Having been an average sized person for the majority of my life, and an overweight person for a regrettable good three years of my life, the ways of the naturally thin have always seemed like a big mystery that managed to elude me. This was especially upsetting because it was not for lack of trying to figure the whole skinny girl magic thing out.

In high school, most of the girls were average sized or a bit overweight. However, there were a few who were embodiments of my ultimate goal – lean, slender and proportional – without seemingly obsessing over their bodies. All the while they ate the same high calorie, junk foods from the cafeteria the rest of us were subjected to, like bagels and cream cheese, waffles, French fries, burgers, and my personal favorite, Philly cheese steak sandwiches with loads of mayonnaise and cheese.

Like everyone else, I know from a young age that I could not eat whatever I wanted and be skinny, given the things I wanted to eat, so I became enthralled with exercise. To me, exercise was the only path to avoid having to give up my favorite foods. While I would putter about in the gym I regularly saw plenty of other average and slightly above average sized girls working out, but for the most part the skinniest girls were not exercise obsessed like the rest of us. I did not know what to make of it, so I chalked it up to their good genes.

In my liberal arts college, waistlines started to expand more and more people weighed on the higher side of average – I guess as a result of the infamous freshman fifteen brought upon by many nights of ramen noodles, pizza and beer pong. However, there were still quite a few enviable bodies strolling around campus in booty shorts and midriff baring tops for me to covet.

Unfortunately, none of my friends fit into the category of hot bodied bombshells, so I had no inside track on how to achieve one of those figures and I remained near the middle of the recommended weight range for my height.

Over the years, the questions still plagued me and the answers still eluded me despite reading weight loss books, articles in magazines, and online forums. Not unlike other women, I can admit to googling how French women enjoy delicious pastries for breakfast while still fitting into their skinny jeans. I have spent an enormous amount of time observing the svelte Japanese women on my multiple trips to Japan, bewildered at how they could eat mounds of rice (i.e. carbs) and still maintain their wide mile thigh gaps, and yes, I too have fallen pray to the click bait promising to reveal the secret to some celebrity's shocking quick weight loss secrets.

The answers to the burning questions in my inquiring mind were never sufficient though. According to these individuals their secrets were being naturally thin, being so busy they forgot to eat, good genes that allowed them to eat whatever they wanted, a high metabolism, hating the taste of chocolate or sweets, or some other anecdote that was seemingly beyond their control.

I begrudgingly bought into every single word until I finally got into the diet and fitness world, became a member of the thin girls club, and befriended other slender, weight conscious individuals. It was then that I finally came to realize what it really takes to get and stay slim like the small group of girls from my high school, the French and Japanese women whom I had admired all those years, and even the secretive celebrities.

I can tell you right now, all that stuff about being naturally thin and hating tasty foods like cake is just as you probably suspected, a load of crap. Seriously, it is nonsense, rubbish, or if we want to really call a spade a spade, complete BS. There is a ton of stuff that the overarching majority of slim people do to have and maintain their banging bodies that is entirely within their control. Unfortunately, a lot of the work, attitudes, and behaviors are things you would never know because it is now taboo to fess up to wanting to be thin, much less making an effort to be.

Thanks to the fat acceptance movement we now live in more than a fat tolerant climate in the United States. Fat acceptance has quickly turned into fat encouragement and fat normalization. According to the Center for Disease Control (CDC), the United States has already rocketed past an obesity rate of one third of the population with an overall obesity rate of 37.9% adults age 20 and older. Additionally, more than two-thirds (70.7

percent) of adults are considered to be overweight or obese. This date is from 2013-2014, and it has only gotten worse since then.

The new trend definitely seems to be that since the majority of people are fat, the solution has been to start brainwashing the populace to accept this as the new normal since it is much easier than fixing the actual problem. In other words, the notion of being skinny and slim is now closely being connected to words like eating disorders and unrealistic.

Of course, that is insane, but the rhetoric seems to be that anyone who wants to be skinny must be doing it under duress from the male dominated hierarchy and media, and admitting to the measures that goes into remaining slim will most definitely make you vulnerable to accusations of not loving or accepting your self – because heaven forbid you might not actually be at optimal health currently and want to do something about it.

The above is why there is such a large disconnect between people who are looking to lose weight and the skinny women they look to for advice on how to replicate their results. Far too many skinny women downplay or lie about what it really takes to have their tight bodies, so when an overweight person actually tries to implement the either incorrect or vague and unrealistic advice touted by skinny girls, they end up falling short and thinking something is wrong with them. In reality, they just do not have the full picture or the whole truth, so of course they do not get the results they are expecting.

That is where this book comes in. I am no stranger to controversy, as evidenced by my best selling books '*The Thigh Gap Hack*', '*Bye-Bye Thunder Thighs*', '*How to Lose Water Weight*', and '*The Easy Diet*' otherwise known as the oil free diet. I do not mind tackling the subjects normally swept under the rug and revel in writing about topics that I would want to read about.

I only wish a book like this existed when I first began to ponder and seek out the answers regarding weight loss that I will be revealing in short order. My life would have been filled with a lot less disappointment from implementing ineffective, foolhardy advice, and I would have reached my goal body a lot faster. I also could have saved a lot of time spent wasted in the gym during high school doing more fun and productive stuff, like spending time with my first boyfriend, and a lot more time in college socializing and having fun than wondering how to stop piling on the pounds. My guess is I am not the only one who would appreciate being leveled with.

To provide you with the intel I will be disclosing very soon, I have turned to my fellow skinny girl friends made up of fitness instructors and trainers, media personalities, models, those who work in the fashion industry, and amazingly fit strangers on the street whom I have interviewed for my YouTube web series called "What's her Secret to that Body?" at www.youtube.com/thighgaphack.

It goes without saying that I have also included my personal experience to round out the lowdown, so we are not talking hypotheticals here. I say all of this to say that you can take the advice within these pages to the bank, because it is coming from a group of individuals that walk the walk.

Just as you would probably want to take hair advice from a stylist with luscious, healthy hair, and dental advice from someone with perfectly straight and white teeth, you should strive to only take weight loss advice from people who have the body you want and have managed to successfully maintain it over the course of time.

That being said, it is important to note getting people to reveal personal habits and secrets is much easier said than done. Not surprisingly, it is much easier to get to the truth when people feel safe from being judged or criticized for caring about their aesthetic, and like they are just trading similar experiences. For this reason, many of these conversations were held off the record and therefore, the names have been changed to protect the innocent.

To be clear, this is not about revealing tips and tricks or behaviors and attitudes of individuals who suffer from eating disorders, mental illnesses, or the like. This is what every day image and weight conscious individuals who do not starve themselves, binge, purge, or abuse weight loss substances do to look amazing in the buff, and how they think to obtain the figure you likely desire to have.

By the end of your reading, you will have unprecedented insight into how to get and stay slim beyond the simplistic advice of eating less and moving more that every single person on the face of this earth has heard a million times before. After that it will be up to you to pick and choose which strategies and ideologies you want to adopt, or you may just decide the effort to be thin is more than you want to or can assume at this time.

Either way, your curiosity will be ultimately satisfied and the guessing game as to how everyone else around you manages to get amazing results, while following their advice to the tee has yet to work for you will no longer be a burning mystery.

The last thing I want to address before we dive in pertains to the title of this book. I am going to preemptively state upfront that all skinny women are not liars, and all skinny women do not lie about all the topics covered in this book. There is no way I can speak for millions of people on the planet, but I can speak on the proven and quite common fabrications and exaggerations many of the folks who belong to this group spread.

My goal is not to malign slim people, a group that I worked my butt off to finally become a part of. We are not bad, duplicitous, or selfishly want to keep our knowledge to ourselves. Again, understand that everyone has a perfectly justifiable reason (at least in their mind) behind the things they do and it is no different in this case.

I will try to shed some light on the thought processes that exist behind many of these lies, but I want to make sure you are not missing the forest for the trees. Keep your eyes on what matters, the prize. In this case, the prize is being privy to what it truly takes to not have to live out the rest of your life in a body you are unhappy with grasping at straws that are guaranteed to get you nowhere. I am handing you the map key to find the hidden doors, so do not focus on anything but the treasure.

Chapter 1 – Dieting

To begin, I want to start off with one of the biggest lies skinny women tell, which is that they do not diet or are not on a diet. Now, as a woman you are probably aware of that fact that tons of women diet, so it seems odd that skinny women would want to conceal this fact.

Well, the first reason very few skinny people ever admit to dieting is because the word itself is now officially taboo. I subscribe to the old definition of the word, which means to eat sparingly or restrict oneself to small amounts or special kinds of food in order to lose weight. The problem is everyone does not seem to agree with this definition.

Unfortunately, more and more people use the word dieting interchangeably with crash dieting, which is a weight-loss diet undertaken with the aim of achieving very rapid results; or yo-yo dieting, which is the cyclical loss and gain of weight. Of course, these are extreme forms of dieting, but it is completely possible to diet without resorting to these measures.

Yet, the fact of the matter is, in today's world dieting is frowned upon. It is associated with harmful extremes and is constantly being touted as not working. Instead, we are encouraged to make an overall lifestyle change or do nothing at all because we should accept and love ourselves the way we are.

However, making a lifestyle change is really no different from dieting since nothing in the definition mentions a specific length of time. If you have come to think of dieting as short term though, then just think of it as something you do over a prolonged period (one's life) and presto, you have got yourself a lifestyle change.

Another defense for dieting is that while the definition mentions special kinds of food, it does not stipulate the specific food one has to eat. Most people do not realize how vague and non-committal the word diet or dieting truly is. Again, people just erroneously associate diet food with franken-foods that have been stripped of their natural fats or qualities to boast a lower calorie number.

Lastly, it bears pointing out that I have nothing against the idea of the overall lifestyle change, which is held in a higher esteem versus dieting and denotes only eating so-called clean, healthy foods. Obviously there is nothing wrong with minimally processed whole foods, but just like some diets can lead people down the rabbit hole of unhealthy eating habits, it can also lead others down the path of enlightened, healthier eating habits.

As for accepting and loving yourself the way you are right now as the catalyst for resisting dieting, what no one ever seems to admit is that it is much easier to love yourself when you are happy with yourself, one aspect of that being your appearance, than not. If you have spent years neglecting your health and body and running it into the ground, finally taking responsibility for what you eat so that you can be happier with your body is a pretty huge display of self-love.

The fact is the most efficient way to lose weight and prudent way to keep it off is with the help of a diet - and we are not talking about unhealthy and extreme starvation diets here. Merely counting calories and/or watching what you eat fits into the definition of a diet. Thus, it makes sense that so many thin people embrace dieting.

Yet, finding a thin person who admits to utilizing this foolproof strategy is a completely different story. Beyond the negative stigma of the word diet, thin women who diet are subject to way more scrutiny, judgment, and criticism than overweight people. If we are being real, it is not uncommon for those who cannot relate or understand why someone with an ideal body is not eating with reckless abandon to immediately jump to accusations of an eating disorder.

In reality, the more obvious explanation is their desire to remain thin, which they know from experience is more akin to a full time job that is necessary to pay the bills than a college internship at your uncle Jimmy's ice cream shop just to get some free credits and spending money – slacking does not cut it. By the way, slacking does not just pertain to junk foods, but just being vigilant about all foods. After all, you can most certainly still get fat from overeating healthy foods, many of which contain an awful lot of calories (avocados, lentils, nuts, and oils being prime examples).

While this may seem like overkill to outsiders, there are countless studies that have shown that people who maintain weight loss over the long term typically make it their top priority. This means they continue to monitor the foods that pass their lips and/or exercise to counteract eating a little more after reaching their goal weight.

The rules of constant awareness and mindfulness are the same for so-called naturally thin individuals who have been skinny all their lives, as well as the nouveau skinny that join the club later in life. When paying attention to your diet no longer becomes a priority, complacency sets in and weight gain almost assuredly follows.

You see, maintaining ones weight requires achieving just the right balance of calories in versus calories out, and that is a really hard task to accomplish in our abundant, food obsessed culture. The second you get complacent and give up tracking, the pounds inevitably start to creep back up thanks to temptations at work, social obligations (e.g. brunch or dinner with friends, celebrations), a bombardment of commercials and marketing from food companies, and even our own friends' social media feeds.

To top it off, we are prone to underestimate the nutritional content of foods and how much we eat, and overestimate how much we exercise - a trifecta of forces that will shrink all the clothes in your closet without ever getting in contact of a washer or dryer. Therefore, actively dieting in an attempt to lose a couple of pounds even when you are already skinny is the best offensive maneuver you can make to continue being a card carrying member of the skinny club.

Being skinny is Easy

Yet another very common reason skinny women lie about dieting that is a bit more sinister than avoiding the negative stigma associated with the word and judgment from presumptuous people, is because they want to misleadingly portray being skinny as easy and effortless.

There is no denying a lot of people aspire to be thin. According to a 2016 Gallup poll, forty nine percent of Americans said they would like to lose weight. However, obesity rates are still on the rise, with about two third of the population being overweight or obese, and only twenty four percent of Americans are reportedly trying to seriously lose weight.

One possible explanation for the huge disconnect is that dropping fat is not exactly a cakewalk. It is a lot easier and more enjoyable to dive into the endless hot breadbasket than to deprive yourself of carbs. Despite general knowledge of the effort necessary to be thin, many women feel jealousy or contempt for those who get or remain skinny through copious amounts of work and self-discipline. In fact, it seems the more effort involved to look a certain way renders the results less valuable.

Maybe those feelings stem from people being reminded of their own shortcomings, or feeling judged – as if the skinny bitch with superior willpower thinks she is cuter and above everyone else. Maybe people think women who prioritize being skinny are vein, shallow, vapid, or trying too hard to seek male approval.

Regardless of the reason, even though the majority of people want to lose weight, women who are living proof that a very narrow kind of perfection really is possible with some sacrifice, are prime targets. I totally get it - when you try to love yourself the way you are but you are unhappy, and you see others choosing what you cannot or chose not to, feelings of resentment and insecurity are likely to surface.

To be clear, it is not just thin dieters that elicit these responses. Those who exercise regularly, which we will talk about later, also raise eyebrows. That being said, dieting more so than exercise seem to signal the green light for detractors to vocalize unsolicited opinions either to each other or worse, to the unfortunate person who happens to be in their crosshairs.

A perfect illustration of this point is oftentimes those feelings of jealousy and contempt is greatly diminished when Mother Nature is blamed for a person's model like physique and ability to defy the law of thermodynamics. That is not to say people who cannot keep weight on no matter how much they claim to try, according to the people who see them pig out regularly, never experience their own share of ignorant comments. However, since their thinness appears to be out of their hands, the vitriol is lessened.

Instead of quips about needing to eat a sandwich, those who witness a thin girl eat a sandwich, bag of chips, and chocolate cake will reason, "Well, she's a carb lover and is still slim because she has great genes. I just have terrible genes, so it's not my fault I'm fat!" In other words, the belief that someone has lucked into thinness makes the belief of being merely unlucky instead of responsible for being overweight more viable.

Celebrities are particularly guilty of touting the "I never diet; I eat what I want and never gain weight" lie to fulfill the dichotomy of the industry pressures to look a certain way while remaining relatable and likable to the every day woman.

The motivation behind their actions is quite understandable, because when Amanda Seyfried says she is hungry all the time to stay in the shape she is and Victoria Beckham confesses to eating very little when she goes out for dinner, they get raked over the coals.

Yet, when women who are rumored to have insured their million dollar bodies like Heidi Klum, Taylor Swift, Rihanna (all of whom have reportedly insured their legs), or the latest it girl wax poetic about loving their junk food but look like they have not touched a burger since entering the limelight, they are celebrated as being normal - although they are definitely not the norm or telling the whole truth.

That is why I find it so refreshing when a brave celebrity pulls back the curtain and dishes out the real scoop. For example, actress Julian Moore has not shied away from talking about the hard work and dieting it takes to look as good as she does on the red carpet; And who can forget when 90210 actress Tori Spelling, who had previously attributed her speedy return to her post baby body on swimming, revealed that was all a farce and that she actually lost the baby weight by cutting down on food.

*"I really don't exercise much, period. So I took my weight off the old-fashioned way. I like to call it the Just Keep Your F***ing Mouth Shut and Eat Air diet. It's all the rage."* – Tori Spelling.

Tori also added that women really did not want to know that she had lost weight through dieting, not exercising, so she simply said that she swam even though she could not do much more than a doggy paddle at the time.

The sad fact is Tori was one hundred percent right. Most women do not want honesty; they want the feel good, fairytale that keeps them implanted in their comfort zone. This brings me back to my earlier point about skinny women merely telling people what they want to hear instead of the truth about their lifestyle and habits. It is the prime example for why a book like this needed to be written and why I am proud to be the one to write it.

Imagine how perplexed and frustrated the mommy desperate to ditch her maternity wear for her old wardrobe feels when she starts swimming to replicate Tori's results and does not get nearly the same outcome. She will likely come to the conclusion that something must be wrong with her, like she is not swimming hard or long enough, or that she is just not destined to be as skinny as she would like, even though that could not be further from the truth. In actuality, she will have failed because Tori omitted a pretty pertinent detail that plays a way bigger role in weight loss than exercise ever could - dieting.

Unfortunately, most celebrities will never reveal the truth behind their enviously hot bods like Victoria Beckham, Tori Spelling, Amanda Seyfried, and Julian Moore. They are more than happy to give interviews raving about their penchant for junk food while sometimes citing Yoga, Pilates, swimming or jet set lifestyles for keeping the pounds off. Of course this is all patently false.

The funny thing about the claims of eluding weight gain despite gorging on fast food is that many of these individuals have photos floating around at some point in their usually earlier career with fuller physiques. These photos are undeniable proof that they are just like us mere mortals who gain weight under the right - or wrong - circumstances.

Nevertheless, by only telling half the story or fabricating the story altogether, the peanut gallery gets to feel less guilty about giving in to the same vices, and subsequently are less inclined to dehumanize and villainize the celeb. It is what is considered a win-win, and why the majority of skinny women will continue to lie about how easy being thin comes.

The Skinny Girl's Diet

After revealing that getting or remaining skinny means dieting like those who are skinny, you may be wondering which diet of choice most elect to follow. Unfortunately, there has been no study conducted on the most popular diet amongst thin women, so no one can say definitively what that is.

What we do know is all skinny women do not follow one specific diet per say, but they know the tenets of the latest and greatest diets like Whole30, the Dash diet, Paleo, juicing, and the classic diets like Atkins, the Mediterranean diet, and The Zone Diet, and basically follow the same principles when they need to reign in a period of over indulging or to look their best for some upcoming occasion.

To be honest, it does not really matter which diet you choose to follow. You can pick one or combine the principles from a few. The most common denominator all these diets share is that they cut down on calories first and foremost.

Some accomplish that by recommending cutting down or cutting out carbs and sweets, while others pinpoint cutting down fat to get the job down. Others utilize fasting, which can be done intermittently (e.g. fasting 8 hours per day every day or fasting two days out of the week, eating one or two meals a day, etc.) to lower the overall calories. Yet and still, other diets recommend only eating whole foods, vegan or vegetarian friendly foods, or fruits.

From personal experience and observations, reducing the number of carbs you consume, following a version of if it fits your macros, and intermittent fasting are the latest most beloved dieting techniques thin girls use because it allows for followers to eat higher volumes of food and blend in with everyone else in social food settings.

For example, if I know I will be attending a three course meal with friends at an event late in the evening, I will refrain from eating anything else the entire day (intermittent fasting) because I know those three courses will amount to my entire calorie allotment for the day. The upside is I can be more flexible with whatever I choose to eat (If it fits my macros).

I will not make any huge declarations, and will still be cognizant of what courses I order, but no one will be giving me the side eye for skipping the appetizer or taking one bite from my dessert, because I will eat it all. The best part is I am spared the criticism without slacking on my diet and all will be well in the world.

The Takeaway

The takeaway from all this dieting talk is that you need to throw out the negative stigma in your head about dieting if you want to lose weight. Seriously, all the skinny girls are doing it in some way or form, even if they claim they are not dieting altogether, or are not following a named program. If you do not want to deal with the negative stigma of dieting, take a cue from the pros and keep your intentions under wraps or call it a lifestyle change if that helps you justify counting calories and cutting down on your food consumption. Whatever floats your boat.

Just know dieting needs to happen because while our metabolism accounts for the largest amount of calories we burn a day, our diets accounts for 100% of our calorie intake, and is the second largest variable in whether a weight loss plan proves successful or unsuccessful.

There is a reason people say you cannot out exercise a bad diet. One grueling hour of exercise can be totally erased with a bag of popcorn or likely your favorite junk food / guilty treat. If you are anything like me, you can inhale a lot of whatever your favorite junk food is in no time flat. Keep eating the way you always have while introducing exercise, while good, will take you ages to get to skinny (and you will probably give up by then), so pick a dieting plan and get started today.

Chapter 2 – Junk Food and Healthy Food

If you were to raid my fridge and cupboards right this very second, you would find a good deal of undeniably healthy foods such as kale, arugula, skinless chicken breast, tuna, cantaloupe, avocados, smoked salmon, etc.

Come back around my birthday and you will find an entire cheesecake from the world famous Junior's Restaurant because it is my favorite dessert, plus a carton of fresh strawberries and whip cream to boot. Check in on a Friday and you may also find a bag of kettle popcorn, ice cream, and my second favorite dessert, macarons (the colorful French desserts, not the coconut cookies).

To be honest, my diet is about eighty percent healthy to twenty percent unhealthy, and at certain times in my life - or the month if we are being real - the numbers shift higher in unhealthy food's favor. While I do not eat rice, bread and pasta, I know a fair share of ladies who do and still remain a size zero. They just may not be enamored or as intensely under the spell of cheesecake, popcorn, ice cream, and macarons. Hey, we all have our different vices.

I am not an anomaly. Skinny women are real people who grew up getting hooked on the same foods you probably did. That beach babe on your body goals Pinterest board is not automatically health conscious by virtue of her flat stomach or lean legs. In fact, her particular diet might be the inverse of mine and consist of twenty percent healthy foods to eighty percent unhealthy foods.

However, the idea that skinny women never stray from the straight and narrow is reinforced all the time. We see it on sites like 'You Did Not Eat That'. You might be thinking, *didn't we just discuss how common it is for celebs and other dieters to exaggerate how much they eat in the last chapter?* Indeed, but we are now talking about when skinny women actually do reach for decadent treats. The big fat lie they will not reveal but I will, is that they do pig out, but as you will soon find out, a little differently than others.

If we are being frank, a woman living in the twenty first century is very unlikely to go her entire life without ever eating something that would nit constitute as a healthy choice. In other words, do not believe for one second that to be thin means being automatically resigned to only eating cabbage, carrots and broccoli, or staring into a dry salad for every meal.

After all, French women manage to stay thin while eating pastries and regularly drinking wine, and Japanese women have consistently been some of the skinniest women in the world without giving up rice, the plethora of Asian snacks, or popular fried dishes. These groups of women do not remain skinny by an unfaltering aversion of life's guilty pleasures. So, how do they do it? The marked difference is in the how we indulge and/or the aftermath of said indulgence.

How Skinny Women Indulge

A few years ago I went to an adult summer camp in Connecticut. In case you are not familiar with the concept, an adult summer camp is where you sleep away from home in bunks with strangers and play sports and silly games in the great outdoors much like you would in regular summer camp.

Unlike regular summer camp, which typically lasts for a few weeks or months, you only stay for a weekend or a long weekend. Another area adult summer camp differs from regular summer camp is that you have all-inclusive access to delicious catered foods and drink, not drab uninspired meals you might normally find in a kids summer camp.

One of the women I met during my time in Connecticut, who we will call Marla, really seemed to embrace this aspect of the camp and every time I would see her, she had some kind of food in her hand. Of course, the only reason her eating habits registered and stood out so much was for the simple fact that Marla was an itty bitty thing.

The very last day of camp, we all watched as she descended from the meal hall with an ice cream Sundae that would rival any calorie bomb monstrosity that might come out of your typical middle American fast casual dining restaurant, like Friendly's or Carvel. This sundae had multiple scoops of ice cream, brownies, cookies, whip cream, candies, and more precariously piled on top. No one thought she would finish the thing, but finish it with much gusto she did.

I happened to become friends with Marla outside of camp and once she returned to the reality of her life, her reckless abandon for food vanished.

However, I happen to know her bunk mate, who was significantly larger and who we will call Jan left in awe of how Marla could give any competitive eater a run for their money while remaining pint sized.

Jan spent a lot of time with Marla and I that weekend but did not remain in our circle of friends outside of camp. She spent three days with Marla seeing everything Marla, and I mean everything. You will understand what I mean if you have ever been in a similar environment. For those who have not, when you find friends at camp it is not uncommon to become inseparable.

Jan left thinking she had a very accurate picture of how Marla normally ate, when in reality that just is not the case. The point is even a weekend is only a small snapshot of time. It is hard for you to get an idea of the amount of food a person is really consuming unless you follow someone around 24/7 over a much longer period of time.

I say all of that to say whereas overweight folks might have junk food every single day, their skinny counterparts are very likely to pig out far less often or only for special occasions before returning to their true eating habits.

At the beginning of this chapter, I listed the snacks you might find in my house on a Friday, but check back any of the other six days of the week and it is a different story. I allow myself one day a week to stray off my diet path; for some girls it may be less (once every two weeks) and for others it may be more (on the weekend). Either way, scarfing down junk food is not a part of our daily routines.

There is a marked difference in ones appetite in general, especially when junk food enters the equation, when you eat poorly all the time versus sparingly. First, the more you feed your sweet or salty tooth, the more you want to continue feeding it, and we all know junk foods usually are very high in calorie and do not leave us feeling satisfied for long.

Secondly, due to the nature of these foods they do not leave you hungry for carrots. You will want more of the same high calorie sweet and savory foods. My friends, that is not a combination of forces you want to contend against.

Granted, indulging only once in a blue moon makes sense, sounds like a great plan, and I am one hundred percent positive you would love to be able to kick your daily bad habits – the problem is, you probably are not sure how. You are in luck, because I am about to share a few of the ways I, and other skinny girls, manage to keep cheat meals and days to a minimum.

First, I want to stress that none of us are super human or have super human willpower. If my favorite food is present and it has been a long time since I have had some, I will likely partake in an unplanned treat. Therefore, I take action to make sure the opportunities do not arise. Simply put, the art of following through on your plan to cut out regular junk food binges is to structure circumstances so that you do not need to rely on willpower.

The first way I cut my willpower some slack is by not bringing my favorite treats and junk food items in my house regularly. When I do feed my cravings, I pick my battle wisely and make sure to only buy one bag of goodies total; so one bag of popcorn, or one box of macarons, never both or multiple bags of my favorite treats as though I am stocking my own supermarket shelf. To be clear, when I say one bag or box, I am not talking the Costco or family pack size bags either; the lower the servings in your treat, or closer you can get to a single serving size, the better.

For me, and many other skinny chicks, it is so much easier to indulge without falling off the diet cliff by making one decision to only buy one treat. This way you never have to wrestle with stopping at bag number one once you have gotten started (remember, eating these foods will usually leave you hungry for the same foods very quickly), and three more bags of goodies are a matter of feet away, because you it will not be possible.

What also lessens the burden of decision-making is shopping infrequently. I typically go grocery shopping once a week and have been trying to stretch that out to once every two weeks. Back before my skinny days, I used to go grocery shopping multiple times a week, and each time my willpower to not buy junk was tested I usually lost.

If you are making multiple stops a week to satisfy your craving for junk resolve now to make a list and only visit the supermarket once a week. Note, this includes corner stores and small shops that sell food, but excludes restaurants and café's.

What makes it easier for me is not carrying any cash or credit cards on me. This ensures I cannot make impromptu stops and have to contend with the devil on my shoulder urging me to pick up an item from the store whenever I pass a marketing message for some yummy looking food. I do keep my credit card details on my person though should I need to pay for something in an emergency. Another awesome benefit of not carrying cash and credit cards is that I am also able to forego eating out at café's and restaurants as well.

Once in my junk food barren kitchen, the likelihood of leaving to make a midnight run isn't happening as parking in my city is sparse and I'm not giving up my spot for anything. Of course, parking might be a cinch in your neighborhood and thusly, it is much easier to run out to pick something up from the store when the thought occurs.

If this is the case for you, ask someone to block your car in your driveway, plan evening engagements that end after your closest grocery store closes, or have someone hide your car keys or take your car until the store closes and you break your habit.

Yet still, if your issue is not so much going less frequently but dealing with temptation once you get to the store, if possible, I would highly recommend you skip the big chain supermarkets altogether and do your weekly or bi-weekly grocery shopping at the farmer's market instead. Not only will you be supporting local farmers and getting fresher produce, you are guaranteed to find less tempting processed snacks like Oreos and Pop tarts to buy.

The marketing departments of these huge corporations spend lots of money for their addictive products to be placed in prime shelf space and ensure their packaging jumps out and beckons you to buy. However, if these are not for sale at all, and you would be hard pressed to find them at farmer's markets, it becomes a million times easier to avoid purchasing. Out of sight, out of mind!

If you find yourself failing miserably at keeping the bad stuff you love out of your cupboard and fridge, consider passing your shopping off to someone else. If you have a spouse, friend, or family member who is healthier, wants to get healthier/lose weight, or just supports you on your journey, ask if they could shop for the both of you.

Perhaps you can alternate weeks where they shop for you and you shop for them. It is not such an absurd idea when you think about it. For instance, imagine your mother asked you to help her lose weight or ditch her unhealthy eating habits and asked you to do all the shopping for her. You probably would not have any trouble sticking to only buying her vegetables, fruits, and lean proteins, and bypassing the soda, cookies, and ice cream that she loves, right? But when it comes to you wanting to lose weight and ditch your unhealthy eating habits you still find it hard to not throw your favorites in the cart.

This is because we tend to be able to apply good advice for others more than we do for ourselves. Oftentimes, it is hard to be your own adviser because you are too close to your own problems, and so your emotions are more likely to cloud your judgment. It is much easier to identify the most rational option, on the other hand, when you have got an outsider's vantage point. Since we know this about human nature, there is no shame in exploiting our natural tendency to reach our desired end goal.

If the last suggestion is unrealistic because you live alone or you are the closest thing to health conscious in your circle, fear not. Everything is for hire nowadays. Take a cue from the elderly and hire folks to do your shopping for you. An added benefit is you will have more free time to yourself.

Draw up a grocery list, hop on Postmates, Taskrabbit, Uber Rush, or any other similar service that deliver goods locally by courier, and pay someone to help keep you on track. Again, doing this is akin to hiring a personal trainer to steer you in the right direction in the gym and there is nothing shameful about being proactive about getting your diet on track. The skinny girl's mindset is to do whatever it takes, be damned. You need to adopt this mindset as well.

Now if you are worried about your wallet, or inconveniencing your friends and family, the good news is this does not have to be permanent. We know it takes about three weeks for a habit to set in, and after phasing out junk foods from your diet over time you will be able to resist it much more readily than when it is firmly a part of your palette.

Prepping

It goes without saying that all thin women are not a monolith, and there is more than one road that leads to the extra-small rack at the retail stores. That being said, there are some girls who will indulge in the fattening, sweet and salty foods we classify as junk more often – even frequently. However, they are doing something their plumper counterparts are not.

I mentioned before my practice of not eating anything all day when I have a social obligation that will involve lots of food, like a dinner reservation or a party. Anyone sitting at the table with me, save for my boyfriend who knows the deal, or observing me from afar might wonder where all the food I can put away on a day like that goes – much like Marla and Jan. That is because they are incorrectly assuming that I have eaten breakfast and lunch on top of what they witness me eating. In reality, it seems like I eat a lot when I am just consuming my normal days worth of calories.

This is a huge departure from what non-skinny people do when they have an event that involves a lot of food. Just the thought of skipping one meal, much more two, might be sending you into a conniption. Except, there is nothing crazy at all about it.

I know that I need to have a certain amount of calories per day to be at my preferred weight (we will talk about the lies skinny girls tell about calories and weight, and how many calories I strive to eat a day soon enough), so when necessary I simply have all of my calories at once instead of broken up over eight or nine hours.

The point is many of the women you see indulging in treats more often also eat fewer meals the majority of the other time, and eat less food in general because junk foods are pretty calorie dense. It is pretty rare to find thin women who practice this because it does require spending a lot of time hungry, but it is not unheard of. Such is the price to pay for eating a lot of unhealthy foods while remaining slim.

One and Done

Another way in which skinny girls indulge differently than the non-skinny is by having a handle on the one and done approach. What is that, you might ask? It is exactly what it sounds like, and you have probably been privy to seeing this technique implemented, much to your disbelief. We are talking about when someone eats treats, but can stop at just one: one cookie, one cupcake, one French fry (or only one handful) – you get the idea.

The picture of the bikini clad girl with visible abs smiling next to a sky-high burger from Carl's Jr., gooey grilled cheese sandwich, or some serious mouth watering pastries might make you scratch your head wondering if she actually gave in to temptation. If she is a one and done girl, it is quite possible she did, just not in the way you would.

A sizable chunk of slender women fit into this category, although they take a lot of heat when someone observes them in practice. There have been exposés written on the prevalence of food bloggers who are accused of misleading readers into thinking they eat everything they post on their platforms while maintaining a good figure.

One of the first and most notable example was an article in Marie Claire written by Katie Drummond that detailed her experience at a weekend long healthy living conference where she witnessed popular food bloggers take hoards of photographs of stacked plates and rave about the amazing food online, despite abandoning their meals after one or two bites. Naturally, insinuations of eating disorders abounded.

When it comes to this controversial topic, it is important to stress that everyone's idea of treating themselves is not the same. As long as a person is not claiming to eat a donut while secretly only licking the powder from the top before chucking it in the trash, there is nothing to be outraged by. It is not her fault people make assumptions that a picture automatically means she will devour the entire thing. Furthermore, if she only chooses to eat half or a couple of bites it need not be overtly stated.

No one is obligated to spell out what he or she eats in a day. Have you ever seen people demand bigger girls disclose exactly how much of a food she has consumed for everyone to dissect? Even if we did require this on both ends of the spectrum, we still would not get a completely accurate picture because interestingly enough, while thin women overestimate how much they eat, larger women do the complete opposite.

Additionally, thin women tend to eat a lot slower than larger women. As everyone knows by now, eating slower allows you to realize when you are actually full faster, as it takes the brain about twenty minutes to register and send out signals to your body. If you still felt hungry and thus kept eating for twenty minutes past the time your belly is full, you can imagine how much extra food and calories a person could unnecessarily consume.

In conclusion, like the person who says she ate so much for the day when compared to someone else she has barely scratched the surface, her perception and experience should not be negated. Nothing is wrong with being able to stop at one bite of Junior's cheesecake. If you can, more power to you! Some people might think it is unnatural or disturbing to not just enjoy the entire treat, when it is really just a form of portion control – something we cannot count on restaurants to do for us in America.

Worth the Calories

If you have been paying attention, by now you know I can count my favorite foods on one hand - popcorn, macarons, and Junior's cheesecake. These are the only foods that I enjoy immensely enough to go to town with. In other words I will not jeopardize my diet for any and every old thing, and if I try something that I immediately do not love, I do not eat it just because it is sugary or just okay – even specific flavors of macarons.

This mindset that myself and other skinny women have, is one where we constantly question whether something is worth the calories or not. Thinking like this is a huge factor in us not eating junk food as often and eating less of it when we do.

You may have heard of this concept in the infamous quote reportedly be uttered by supermodel Kate Moss, "Nothing tastes as good as skinny feels," What this quote means is that nothing – or to some thin women, very little – tastes so good that you over do it and jeopardize your thinness.

If you are struggling with wrapping your head around the concept because you have never been skinny, this is also a decision you can make. Simply think about how you usually feel after eating too much junk food or straying from your diet yet again. I would venture a guess it is not a good feeling. Now, think of how you would feel hitting your goal weight or fitting into your goal outfit, or looking at your ideal naked body in a mirror. That would feel pretty damn good right?

Every time you are tempted to over eat junk food, pause for a moment and contemplate whether it is really worth the calories to feel off track, bloated, stuffed, and out of control, yet again. Does that food you are thinking about eating even taste that spectacular? I would say, even if it is your favorite and you determine it is worth the calories, just having this question in the back of your mind when you are tempted to eat more will stop you from doing so more often than not.

The Aftermath

The above are just some of the ways the thin crowd treat junk food differently than the average overweight or obese American, and the prime reason they do not look like the average American. However, you would be hard pressed to get this information from the horse's mouth.

When talking to people who are not already in the skinny club (and sometimes with those who are also members), the extent of the dialogue often stops at, "I never eat junk food," or "I eat junk all the time and never gain weight". As we now know, both are extremes that are simply not true or truly not that simple.

Equally as important to how we indulge differently, is how we react when we do go a tad overboard versus regular folks – or as I like to call it, the aftermath. The first difference amongst skinny women who may have a larger than normal or desired calorie day, is there is no throwing in the proverbial towel, or spiraling into a sea of shame that involves eating more junk foods, which is the unfortunate reaction of many overweight individuals who diet.

Instead, the skinny girl gets right back on her horse. She might work out extra hard or attempt to be more active that day or the rest of the week to combat the effects as fast as possible. If she is not a big fan of exercise, she might elect to eat a lot less over the next few days so that by the end of the week, the calories will have evened out to a normal week's intake. Either way, overdoing it a bit is not seen as the end of the world or a sign of failure; the next day it is back to business as usual.

A little Bit of Magic

Last, but not least, another way in which we deal with the aftermath of a junk food bender is through a little bit of magic, which I am sad to say bigger girls are not privy to. Every human body wants to maintain equilibrium, so when a thin girl eats a lot more than she normally would, her body will automatically elevate her metabolism and energy levels to combat the sporadic indulgence. It is a secret many women do not even know about, so it is not a big fat lie per say – but it is something everyone definitely does not have in their toolbox.

Do not get be wrong – if even the thinnest girl eats enough pound cakes and burgers frequently enough, her body will not keep self adjusting in this manner forever. Pretty soon it will try to maintain the new, higher set point and the weight stays put.

The only way to experience this phenomenon is to get lean, so you cannot implement this tactic by choice. However, you now know this boost that no one really talks about is one reason many women who should seemingly be gaining weight when they let loose do not, while your experience is not quite the same. Do not worry though, keep unearthing the ways of this secret society and you will be benefitting from a little bit of magic too.

Let's Talk About Taste

Keeping in line with lies about junk and healthy foods skinny women tell, another rampant one you might not find hard to believe is not exactly the truth, is the claim to dislike the taste of junk foods, or love the taste of healthy food more. The reason this idea is not very believable to the majority of vegetable avoiding, fast-food loving individuals is because we all know what junk foods taste like.

To be clear, junk foods are designed by scientists to be highly palatable, or in layman's terms, deliberately addictive. Some of the world's smartest people spend absurd amounts of time tinkering with flavors, textures, smells, etc., probably in a super sophisticated lab, in an attempt to fashion food that is irresistible and down right addictive.

They do so by knowing the markers and desires we all share that many of us are not even consciously aware of. That being said, you better believe the cheesy, sweet, deep fried, and crunchy foods you would eat yourself into oblivion if you could, are just as appetizing to the 100-pound gal as it is to the next person.

On the flip side, if you have visited any of the vegan, vegetarian, raw food, etc. restaurants that are cropping up every day, it would seem safe to say there are plenty of tasty healthy foods that rival junk food. In reality, most of these dishes in the healthy food spots that taste ridiculously good rely on the addition of oils, dried fruit, high calorie avocado and nuts, dressings, etc. to make them more appetizing.

If we are talking about whole foods it just is not possible. Case in point, no one actually thinks baked chicken, boiled sweet potato, or an apple tastes better than fried chicken, sweet potato fries, and apple pie. No one.

Now, although we cannot truthfully deny junk foods objectively taste better than healthy foods, it is possible to convince ourselves we are not huge fans, and that is what thin women are actually going on about. The phrase "I don't like the taste of junk food," really means through a combination of reasons such as: lessening the sensitivity to them (eating them less), knowing how bad it is for you (education), not thinking it is worth the calories (being selective), and having pretty good alternatives (tasty healthier foods), most thin women are no longer slaves to the stuff. Force-feed them a pizza though and they will not be gagging from the repulsive taste.

Another thing worth mentioning is that as previously discussed, living in this modern day and age it is impossible to not eat any junk food, ever. Like superman, every thin woman has her kryptonite. Those who really are not drawn to sweets due to genetics or more exposure to one flavor in their diet while growing up, are sure to derive pleasure from salty snacks like chips, pretzels, or French fries and vice versa.

Even the women who advocate eating clean are sneaking in junk foods by substituting the ingredients and paleo-fying it. You see them sharing recipes with one another for "clean" ice cream made from bananas or soy, brownies made from beans, and cookies made from nut flours and sugar substitutes, etc.

Sure, they might be making these treats in their kitchen instead of getting their fix from a fast food restaurant on the corner, or they may be buying Amy's Organic brand of mac of cheese instead of some generic inorganic brand with a neon colored cheese type substance, but often times these foods have just as much calories as their contemporary equivalent, and/or taste similar to boot.

This is great news for those of you who struggle with dieting because the thought of never eating your favorite comfort foods again depresses you more than anything, but the women with great bodies insinuate it is par for the course. Now you know that none of them have given up every single guilty pleasure in order to get the bodies they have, and you do not have to either.

That being said, by no means am I suggesting you should not curb your junk food habits if you want to get your body snatched. When I first began to lose weight I had to cut back and cut out some items from my repertoire. I used to love McDonald's apple pies and KFC's potato wedges, but since I was cutting out fried foods and desserts that were not worth the calories I stopped considering these places as dining options. It is easy to avoid eating anything from McDonald's, Burger King, KFC, or any other major fast food chain now because over time I have forgotten the taste.

Similarly, you need to make those choices and implement all the other strategies we have just covered to keep the rest of the stuff at bay. Shape your environment so that you are not being tempted and it is not easy to slip up: Clean out your fridge and pantry, go grocery shopping less often or giving someone else the responsibility, forego carrying around money just in case you want to make an unplanned trip to the store, prep for indulgences, deal with slip ups by jumping right back on track, be selective, and question whether the food you are thinking about eating is worth the calories.

Chapter 3 – The Sweat Life

When it comes to exercise there are two common lies skinny women tell. The first is that they never exercise or lead very sedentary lives and still manage to look amazing, and the second is that they exercise all the time because they just love it so much and if they missed a day they would feel incomplete!

We will start with the former idea because I think that is the camp that those who are trying to get skinny are curious about the most since exercise seems to be a unfortunate truth for the majority of people who want to stay on the skinnier spectrum of the BMI chart.

To begin, I would like to recount a recent conversation I had with a teeny tiny member of my boyfriend's soccer team, who we'll call Jane, about how she stayed so slim. As you can probably guess given the nature of this chapter, Jane claimed she "hated exercise," and "never really worked out." Now, anyone desperate to figure out the skinny mystique might just take her word at face value and gripe about her just being one of those mystical lucky girls with an amazing figure.

Given the fact that I know this is a big fat lie many skinny women tell, and since I knew we had just played a forty-five minute game of soccer in which we ran back and forth across a regulation sized field nearly non-stop (we only had the bare minimum number of female players on our team and did not have the luxury of relying on a sub), I pressed deeper. At the very least, I knew she at least regularly got one form of exercise weekly, negating her "I never exercise" claim.

Unsurprisingly, a few minutes later Jane started talking about another soccer team she was on, that she wanted me to consider joining. Instantly, I made a mental note that she was going to do another gruesome workout in a matter of days. Since the context of her revealing this to me was to recruit me, she was probably going to also burn a crap ton of calories because of their lack of subs. As I am sure you would agree, two forty-five minute high intensity workouts per week is a far cry from never working out.

For example, a forty-five minute jog burns a decent amount of calories, but you would definitely not mistake what we had done with jogging. We were sprinting back and forth across a regulation soccer sized field, stopping and turning on a dime, and defending and fighting for the ball. Yet in her mind, she never really exercised.

I could stop there, but Jane is just such a prime example of why you cannot take the "I never exercise" trope at face vale, I will continue. I later on would come to learn that she was a nanny for two very young toddlers, so you know what that means? Her full time job consisted of bringing two high-energy kids to the park, playing with him, cooking for them, cleaning up after them, and much more tasks that are too long to fully list here. As any mother can attest to, taking care of two young children is not exactly a cakewalk, especially when it is your job to play or entertain them and you cannot exactly just give the kid a toy, stick them in front of the television, and opt out. This is why most people try to have kids when they are young and can still keep up with them.

If we add everything up (and I would not doubt there is more evidence we could find that disproves her no exercise stance), all that regular activity rivals and probably exceeds the typical girl with a gym membership taking a dance class three times a week and working a desk job. Yet, if you let Jane tell it, she is a couch potato compared to the gym membership holder. Can you imagine what else she might be doing that she is not calling exercise, but clearly is?

As an aside, I should mention that eating patterns obviously make a huge difference in how much you need to exercise to remain thin. It just so happens that our little soccer group ended up going out to eat at a BBQ joint a short while after, and I could not wait to see what Jane would order. Working out as much as she does, she could get away with a larger meal – which of course would leave everyone else wondering where she put the food.

For dinner, Jane ordered a small side and a beer after revealing she was a vegan. In light of all the information and the full picture, it really is no mystery why Jane has the incredible body she does. It is just too bad that the story she tells others is not quite reality.

I say all of that to say, just because someone does not call all the activity they do exercise, it does not mean they are not exercising. Anything that expends a lot of energy on a daily basis (which is the goal of exercise for weight loss) is undoubtedly exercise. In reality, our aforementioned subject burns enough calories that would rival the most devoted gym rat.

All you need to do is dig a little deeper and ask a few questions about someone's hobbies and/or job, look at their lifestyle and mannerisms (high energy people that cannot seem to keep still probably burn a lot of calories without ever needing to step foot inside a gym), and you will soon realize they do not have great bodies from being sedentary couch potatoes all day.

Workout Love

On the opposite end of the spectrum, an exaggeration notorious in skinny circles is a devout love for exercise. Undoubtedly you have heard of people talk about having to work out, as though if they did not they would suffer severe physical or psychological repercussions. Then there are those who seem to do nothing else but work out all the time, doing two or three hour long sessions and again blaming it on how good it makes them feel.

Hearing this might make you think something is wrong with you for dreading your measly one hour workout two or three days a week. Do not beat yourself up just yet because I have got news for you - none of the skinny chicks that rave about loving exercise so much they never skip a day or do two back-to-back soul cycles classes are telling the truth.

To be clear, they may not be exaggerating about never skipping a workout day - I worked out five days a week without fail for an entire year, but the driving force was not my love for sweating. In fact, I oftentimes had to psyche myself out to get through a session

If we are talking about dance or some other sport with an element of physical activity to it (e.g. fencing or soccer), it is plausible to think love enters the equation. Such activities are not as mind numbing as running or pedaling in place for an hour and could seemingly result in excitement to do that activity.

However, to think a person will love doing even a sport or activity they have a passion for every day or every time is misguided. Everyone has moments of dread, moments where they would rather stay in bed than attend an early-morning workout, or days when they end up cutting their workouts short because they are just not feeling it.

For the majority of people – even thin ones – exercise is a practical means to an end. It is done to burn more calories than ingested, to help reach a specific weight goal, or to pre-empt or counter a particularly bad day or night of eating and drinking. It is not really a preferred pastime activity.

More accurately, what anyone who says they love exercise really loves are the results. They also love the sense of support or community they get from workout dates with friends instead of lunch dates and like-minded people in their classes. The success of places like Soul Cycle and The Barre Method are a testament to this, but even fitness fanatics who go to chain gyms feel part of the larger fitness community when they see regular faces on the floor. The same thing goes for those who play a sport as part of a team or club, or partake in running groups.

Why is it so important to point out the distinction? Again, to think that your lack of an unflinching enthusiasm for exercise makes you a failure compared to your skinny peers is ludicrous. Do not feel too bad about your proclivity to want to make up excuses when leg day rolls around, phone it in for a yoga session, or really push yourself to pop in an exercise DVD. You are not alone, nor are your endorphins broken or anything like that.

In actuality, the hype about endorphins being released during a work out as the catalyst for people exercising like addicts because of the high (e.g. runner's high and yoga bliss) still does not stop dread from creeping in or represent an unconditional love of doing the actual deed. After all, endorphins do not translate from the end of one session to the start of the next – and we all know starting is the hardest part.

The Real Deal

Given we have established thin people struggle with sticking to their workouts too, you may be wondering how they overcome it in the absence of a strong motivator such as love. We will discuss in more detail what does push them and how you can be motivated by the same things they are shortly, but first let's discuss why people lie about this in the first place.

There is no denying fitness is often hailed as the paramount of perfection, attractiveness, and appeal, if you could lose a few pounds. If you are already thin and working out all the time though, people get nervous that you are overdoing it and have a problem.

Even if there is nothing shady going on besides wanting to maintain her figure or reach her specific goal with the help of exercise, she is judged. Therefore, if she says she derives pleasure from exercise or her love for working out prevents her from staying away to no avail, it becomes justified. To illustrate my point, no one would dare tell the ballerina she practices way too much because it is socially acceptable to put in insane hours when it comes to your passion. Take a woman with the same physique as her dedicated to the elliptical machine and suddenly everyone is concerned.

Again, the reason I am highlighting this topic is because it leaves overweight people feeling guilty that they do not love exercise the way they think they should. That being said, you have to understand that this is not an excuse to put off workouts or only focus on diet (although exercising is not mandatory to be skinny it definitely helps and creates a toned shape that most women prefer). Instead, I want you to realize that it is human to feel the way you do, everyone does, but as humans we have been blessed to be able to put our mind over matter.

Pushing Past the Feeling

The fact is true strength begins between the ears and mental toughness, or grit, allow you to persevere when the love is missing in action. We are not talking about relying on motivation; we are talking about forming habits. Once you get yourself into a routine that commits you to your training, you will get going whether you are in the mood or not.

I would add that psyching yourself up is a huge part of mental toughness. Think of the trainers at fitness boot camps who holler and hoot, "You can do anything for 60 seconds!" It seems amazing that simply telling oneself how much you love exercise or have ten more in you, makes it much easier to will yourself to do it, and how telling yourself *"I can't do this,"* will lead you to give up on the spot. It is the good old fake it until you make it strategy. As with every other area of life, attitude and what you tell yourself is everything.

Whereas those who are overweight will admit to not enjoying exercise and therefore be less inclined to push themselves to even begin - much less complete a workout, a skinny person will psych themselves out with the story that they actually enjoy or love running, lifting weights, kickboxing, etc. Logically, if you tell yourself you enjoy doing something there is less of a chance that you will skip it, so here is your permission to lie like the skinny girls and convince yourself that you love working out as much as they do.

Another recommendation to pair with getting your mind right, which makes psyching yourself up easier, is to sample a wide array of workouts and see which one(s) you do enjoy. Getting a Classpass™ membership if it is available in your area helps, or alternatively you could sign up for a gym that offers a variety of classes so if you get tired of the stair climber you could switch to Zumba™. When Zumba™ becomes old news, TRX™ might start calling your name.

A budget friendly option to burn calories without exchanging any money is through workout videos online. Try Pilates one day, cardio kickboxing the next, etc. Between YouTube™, workout challenges, Pinterest™ guides, and all the other websites out there, you could probably do a different workout every single day for free if you wanted to.

If it helps, do not call it a workout like my friend, Jane. Join a soccer, lacrosse, boxing, or swimming team. There are many companies, like Zogsports™, that offer social recreational sports leagues throughout the United States. I am positive they have some competition in your state. Generally, we get excited about new things so keep your workouts fresh and new and you will deal with feelings of skipping less and less. Find a couple of things you enjoy or have interest in trying if you are not sure you enjoy it yet, and rotate to avoid becoming bored and disenfranchised with working out altogether.

Once you find a few activities that stick the next step is to try to become part of a community or multiple communities if you have the time. I get bored out of my mind with running, but long jogs and power walks with my boyfriend make getting my cardio in much more bearable. I push myself to go to my yoga dates with my workout buddies because I know they are expecting me to show up. My sweaty Saturday cardio group gets me out of bed at 8:30 am without fail because I love that crew and if I am not there, I will feel an unshakeable sense of FOMO (fear or missing out). You need to get there as well.

If you currently do not have any friends to do these things with, befriend the people you meet in class. It is surprising how your gym or studio can start to feel a lot more like home if you just start saying, "Hello." and "See you next class!"

Lastly, I want to stress the importance of not overdoing the whole working out thing. This includes non-exercise related activity that technically burns just as many calories as any conventional workout. Overdoing it is a surefire way to burn out and associate negative thoughts with the act. You may be tempted to overdo it when you hear of other woman spending hours in the gym – the thought of becoming addicted yourself might even seem appealing, because then you would not have to deal with convincing yourself to do what needs to be done.

In actuality, research tells us that exercise addiction only affect a very small subset of people – those who exercise when injured or exhausted or exercise to the point what it adversely affects their work or relationships. Sports scientists would classify *healthy* thin women who work out hard and often, but responsibly, as committed exercisers. These people know when to rest, and understand the importance of balance. What is the point in being thin if you are too sick and exhausted to enjoy it?

Chapter 4 – Good Genes

In a recent article detailing how famous pop singer Adele shed her weight, a diet based on eating foods such as kale, berries, capers, cocoa powder, green tea, and turmeric, that supposedly activated her skinny gene (SIRT1) was credited. This skinny gene is said to protect one's cells during times when food is limited or unavailable, inhibits fat storage, and increases metabolism in an effort to promote survival.

The article then went on to mention that her diet involved restricting her calories to 1,000 a day in the first phase, and then 1,500 calories in the second. I could not help but laugh, because this sums up the entire skinny gene argument beautifully.

Obviously there was no mystical skinny gene involved. Adele simply ate a lot less than she normally did, so she became smaller over time. Sadly, tons of people have jumped on this diet bandwagon convinced they too could activate their apparently dormant skinny gene when all they are doing is losing weight the good old-fashioned way of consuming fewer calories.

When it comes to the idea of genes being responsible for our size, it is important to note that DNA does not equate to your destiny. Genes only provide the potential and rely on instructions for what to do, and where and when to do it. For example, a human liver cell contains the exact same DNA as a brain cell, yet it knows to code only those proteins needed for the functioning of the liver.

Those instructions are found not in the letters of the DNA itself but on it, in an array of chemical markers and switches, known collectively as the epigenome, which help switch on or off the expression of particular genes. This fact makes the epigenome just as critical as DNA to the healthy development of an individual.

Yet, the widely perpetuated idea of skinny or good genes as the catalyst for some of the most admirable physiques persists. It is by far one of the biggest lies skinny women tell, but conversely those on the outside looking in also fan the flames of this tale. We see this when thin women say they eat a ton, and/or never exercise, and when larger women say they barely eat and exercise all the time but remain overweight.

It is tempting to assign credit to someone's DNA or genes for a great body begotten by unconventional methods (high calorie diets and no exercise). After all, normal folks with presumably average or regular genes would blow up like a house.

Additionally, all the talk about natural set points, (a set point is the weight range in which your body is programmed to function optimally and set point theory holds that one's body will fight to maintain that weight range), and the correlation between obese people coming from families where a lot of the members are also obese starts to build what some might call a convincing argument. In actuality, it is easy to believe this lie not because the argument is convincing, but because the answer is easy and does not require further delving.

When something happens that we cannot quite explain, we like to chalk it up to magic, super natural powers or superior attributes. For example, we tell little kids Santa Claus is able to deliver gifts to millions of people in one night because of his supernatural flying reindeers and they buy it. It is not just kids though; adults explained droughts and natural disasters on angry gods until we knew better.

While it is easy to think the seemingly miraculously skinny must owe their figures to something mere mortals do not possess, signifying that they are somehow destined to be that way, we now know better.

The first thing we now know is the majority of those perpetuating the theory possess glaringly obvious biases and financial motives. For example, it behooves the people touting the diet Adele supposedly utilized to have people believe there is a skinny gene because their diet is all about activating this gene. According to them, your skinny gene will remain buried and nonfunctional until you buy into their program.

We also know better when it comes to the body. All people have essentially the same 20,000 genes that determine our species. Half are inherited from your mom and half from your dad. You are determined by the combination of genes you inherit, the gene variants in them, and the environments that you expose them to.

I will concede that some women have a tougher hill to climb when it comes to getting as thin as they would like. Our small genetic variations influence differences such as hair color, susceptibility to disease, and weight gain and loss. To be clear, the genes that determine a person's ethnicity (e.g. Asian) will not make them skinny – contrary to popular opinion. We know this because there are clearly larger Asian people in this world (mainly when they get to America and are exposed to the American diet and portions).

Genes play a very small role in your weight, with experts putting the figure at about 25%. This means that being fat, even if you think you are loaded up with all the wrong genes, is by no means a done deal. Let's say due to your genes you have more muscles or are taller, then you will probably be able to eat more food without packing on the pounds since these two factors will allow you to burn more calories than a shorter, less muscular individual.

There has even been research conducted that suggests tall nations are more genetically likely to be slim. That being said, there were low percentages found between genetic variations in height and BMI, and that suggests that environmental factors are actually the main determinant of a nation's BMI.

Additionally, if we look at the opposite of the idea of a skinny gene – a gene that causes obesity, it does not make much sense since no gene could spread through the populations as fast as the rapid increase in rates of obesity since the 1970's, even if it were advantageous (and it clearly is not). It takes a much longer period than five, ten, or even twenty years to see genetic profiles change amongst generations.

It is only since that time that the march of fat has accelerated. Might I add that for some reason this genetic wave does not seem to be present in developing countries. This leads one to question whether all these people in western society have activated their fat gene or is it more likely that more folks are fatter now due to our moving in from the fields, working in sedentary office jobs, having more access to cheaper and more calorific foods, and spending more of our free time on the internet or watching Netflix?

The answer seems quite obvious – genes are not the reason large swatches of people have gotten larger over time. That is the bad news for anyone who has used their bad gees to blame a body they may not be happy with, and the skinny women who has used their good genes to mask the effort it truly takes to be skinny. The good news is that you can influence your genes to an extent by taking control of your environment and turning certain genes off or on.

Even in studies that support the idea of fat genes, like the one from Cambridge University that analyzed more than 50 studies of people with one particular obesity gene and used data relating to more than 200,000 people in several countries, researchers found people carrying the gene had a 30 percent less chance of being overweight if they simply became physically active.

The reason this work is because genes cannot distinguish whether the environmental cues are good or bad for you. They will just react to each stimulus to sustain short-term survival. A perfect illustration of this idea is finding one thin person with your particular ailment or bad luck gene that you contribute to being overweight.

The most common offenses I hear are hyperthyroidism, stomach ulcers, diabetes Crohn's disease, and leptin deficiency. You are bound to find someone else managing their weight despite their genes or disease by controlling their environment. Doing so removes the common held belief and excuse that we are slaves to our genetic makeup and that we really can make a difference simply by changing our behavior.

Once you have disproven the idea you can start to identify stop telling your own big fat lie that many larger women believe – that you have bad genes. Even if you are not a foot taller than other women with more musculature, and thereby not burning as many calories as the glamazon model on the cover of Vogue, just knowing other women your age and size can manage to work with their genes should put you on the right track.

Chapter 5 – The Magic Number

Upon reading the title of this chapter and realizing it pertains to skinny women lying about their weight, you might wonder which woman *doesn't* lie about their weight? I would be inclined to agree with you that most people are not forthcoming about the number they see when they step on the scale, particularly women. As a teenager, for a while there I thought all women were around 120 pounds, since that was the weight it seemed like every model, actress, and singer claimed to be.

The studies affirm what we believe to be true, with one study claiming that two thirds of women have lied about their size, on average reducing their weight by nine pounds. I have a sneaking suspicion that number jumps a lot higher when we look at online dating profiles. These lies have no bounds either, with researchers finding millions of women fib about their weight to their doctor, partner, best friend, the DMV, and even their mother.

So, why is it so important to highlight when skinny women lie about their weight if everyone is doing it? So many normal women lie about their weight, we really do not have a good idea about what accurate/realistic weight and height looks like. Going back to the purpose of this book, it is important to peel back the curtain and bring a dose of reality to the conversation often not seen by anyone who is not already in the skinny club. When those who want to fast track their membership take these untruths at face value, it leads to confusion, frustration, disappointment, and warped expectations.

To start, there are different kinds of fabrications skinny women tell when it comes to weight. The first one you might hear is that she does not know or care about how much she weighs. While all skinny women are certainly not stepping on the scale every single day, for the most part a thin woman knows how much she weighs and monitors fluctuations with the eye of a eagle.

She probably has a number in her head that if she gets close to sounds off alarms and forces her to rein her diet in and/or ramp up her exercise. If there is not a specific number, she knows what that number looks like on her frame in the mirror and feels like in her clothes.

The reason for dodging this question with a nonchalant reply is to ward off judgment, haters, and not come across as being too pleased with her body in a world full of people mostly insecure about theirs. Can you see a pattern forming here?

Generally, it is fine if other people think you look great, but the moment a woman agrees and also starts believing the hype, she must be taken down a few pegs and put back into her place. It may seem pessimistic, but unfortunately, it is the truth and the reason why so many thin women do everything in their power to take the focus off their bodies by dodging the question.

That same desire to take the spotlight off their bodies is also why many thin women lie about their weight in a completely different way most women do. While others are busy subtracting nine pounds from her actual weight, really thin women are known to tack on a few. Seems absurd, but it happens all the time.

It is not that the skinny woman is ashamed of her weight or wants to be bigger, for she typically had to work very hard and exercise a ton of discipline to get to where she is. Again, not everyone can appreciate that or respects her decision to want her body to weigh or look a certain way, so she may round up a few pounds to skirt interrogation or scrutiny and be more in line with what society deems acceptable.

This is akin to saying you eat 1200 calories per day, when you actually eat 1100. A 100-calorie different is not a big one, but society perceives one number to be a healthy amount and another as a starvation diet.

Of course by telling others she is heavier than she actually is, other women who seek to look like her are already operating from an incorrect benchmark and are disappointed when they get to that weight but still look nothing like the person they based their goal on.

This is why I recommend foregoing asking altogether. If you cannot see the person stepping on a scale for yourself, it truly is pointless to ask others how much they weigh, since you will rarely get the truth.

Never Satisfied

Despite her small frame, the skinny woman is only human and like every other human being is never completely satisfied. Sure, most women would kill to have her body, but she already has her body and there is always something that she will be working on (typically her abs or thighs).

Therefore, another lie skinny women tell is that they are no longer trying to watch their weight. I have said it before in other books, but I do not think I have ever met anyone, skinny women included, who was not trying to lose at least five pounds or look more toned. You can probably relate. If we are being real, even the biggest fat acceptance proponents who claim to love their bodies, always seem to proudly appear a few pounds lighter a few years later. See Amy Schumer, Melissa McCarthy, Monique, Roseanne, and the list could go on and on.

Having a constant incentive is a major part of the reason she is able to maintain her thinness. After all, it is no secret that people tend to overestimate how many calories they burn and underestimate how many calories they eat. Thus, when people are trying to maintain their weight it is no surprise that they gain a little instead.

It is like the shark analogy, where the shark must stay in constant motion or die. It is very hard to eat at a perfect equilibrium so that you are consuming just as many calories as you are burning and are therefore maintaining your weight. In actuality, if you are not burning less than you eat, you are burning more and are either losing a little bit of weight or gaining a little bit of weight.

That being said, by always having a goal – whether it be to lose five pounds or tone up a little bit more, the skinny woman does not get complacent and lax enough to be steadily gaining and therefore does not pile on the pounds.

Fudging the Numbers

Lastly, some of the two thirds of women subtracting a few pounds from their actual number is comprised of those you would think do not have any pounds to spare. Particularly, if the thin woman fluctuates within a few pounds, she will most likely default to the lower end of the spectrum even if she knows she is closer to the higher end at the time.

This happens because we all have a number, usually our lowest weight, where we were most pleased with our bodies, and where we would ideally remain. Additionally, women have lied themselves into a corner, saying we weight so little that no one really understands a woman of a certain height and body type can weight more than a certain amount of pounds and still look slender and smoking hot.

That being said, we feel the need to say we are lighter to meet some arbitrary confines. It does not help that the mentality is one of, no harm, no foul. As we know, it is a pretty natural occurrence amongst the majority of women to fudge the numbers without it being perceived as a big deal or hurting anyone, so people will indulge the fantasy and go lower.

Honestly, unless your weight needs to be revealed for a medical or safety related reason, it truly is no one's business. Just as you probably would prefer to keep that number to yourself, so do women who you think should want to shout theirs from the rooftops.

Chapter 6 – Fast Metabolisms

If I had a dollar for every time someone cited a fast metabolism as the reason for being thin, or someone else being thin, I have no doubt I would have a prime spot on Forbe's top list of the obnoxiously rich. The majority of the population, which includes the skinny and non-skinny alike, seem to love this gross over exaggeration, or what I like to call, big fat lie.

The difference between this lie and others though is I have a sneaking suspicion those who buy into the super metabolism idea actually might believe it. After all, it is entirely possible that people just do not know any better and are repeating what they have heard or been told for ages, because this idea is so prevalent in our society despite being patently false.

That being said, the idea of having a fast or overactive metabolism is along the same lines of attributing good genes to a woman's waistline and thigh circumference. Neither is primarily responsible for women's thinness, but besides these perceptions being untrue, it is dangerous. The danger of course, is when you assign all power to a magical metabolism you simultaneously take away the power of people's own effort and get left with people who feel helpless or destined to be fat, and deem trying to be futile.

Like good genes, a super metabolism is just a convenient, kind of lazy, way to explain why someone who eats like a horse and gives Al Bundy a serious run for the title of biggest couch potato, stays thin. If you really think about it, it is a little gullible to believe a magical metabolism alone can give you the perfect little body.

Still, the metabolism excuse is kept alive because it has loads of people with a vested interest in preventing it from dying, so the facts can often get blurred with fiction. We are talking about weight loss clinics, those selling pills, shakes, teas, foods, and even books meant to speed up the metabolism. Finally, it is quite difficult to prove or disprove someone has a fast metabolism, so people just go with it.

Unfortunately, contrary to what any thin person claims, just as good genes is not the main reason the overwhelming majority of skinny women are in fact skinny, super charged metabolisms is also not the scapegoat so many people think it is. Want some proof? Gladly!

First, we need to make sure we are on the same page about what metabolism is and is not. In scientific terms, metabolism is the building up and breakdown of compounds by specific enzymes through biochemical reactions to create energy in order to sustain life. It is regulated by the hypothalamus, which is situated in the lower part of your brain.

The hypothalamus also directly controls hunger, thirst, body temperature, and energy production, which are all important aspects of metabolism. Heart rate is not a direct reflection of metabolic rate – and contrary to what many people think, a lower resting heart rate is considered healthier than a higher one, according to the American Heart Association.

In case I lost you there, in a nutshell our bodies use calories to keep the lights on — our heart needs the energy to pump blood, our lungs need energy to enable us to breathe, our body temperature needs to be maintained, compounds need to be moved in and out of cells, and a bunch of other normal body processes you rarely need to think about has to occur. Yes, we are all high maintenance so to speak, calorically.

So, if you were to lie down on the couch all day long, your body would naturally still burn a fair amount of calories handling these processes. This is called our resting metabolic rate. This is our greatest component of calorie burn, responsible for 60 – 75 percent of the total calories burned each day.

Along with the calories we burn through exercise, bouncing your leg while sitting, walking and digesting food, it makes up what most of us refer to simply as our metabolism. Without metabolism we would lack the energy to get out of bed in the morning, let alone burn calories all throughout the day.

Can you raise your metabolism by drinking ice-cold water, ramping up your caffeine intake, and building more muscle? Absolutely. I talk these tricks of the trade and more in my book, *The Thigh Gap Hack*. That being said, you will not become a calorie-burning furnace and shrink down to the size of your favorite celebrity as a sole result.

Gaining one pound of muscle will only increase your metabolism by approximately five calories, and consuming more caffeine and chili peppers will boost your metabolism for thirty minutes before returning to where it started. So, neither of these factors are going to leave you with a magically souped up increase to rival that of the women claiming to have a magical and enviable rate of metabolism.

I can say this assuredly because in actuality skinny individuals almost invariably have a lower resting metabolism than heavier individuals, since there is literally less of them to burn while at rest. That is right, chances are you are torching way more calories, and as a result have a much higher metabolism, than your skinny friends.

Do not get me wrong, we are all not burning the exact same amount of calories – some people do have slightly faster metabolisms than people who are similar in age and stature to themselves, but overall, people of the same height, weight, and stature generally have the same metabolisms. When skinny folks say they have a fast metabolism, they are insinuating that they burn more calories than other people with all other things being equal. However, it is extremely rare for one's metabolism to be faster, or slower for that matter as seen in metabolic disorders, than normal.

You can prove my point for yourself the next time someone claims to have a really fast (or slow) metabolism by asking that person if they have ever had their metabolism checked. It is safe to say those making the claims will not have done so, yet the only way one would know whether they have a very fast metabolism, relative to other people their age, weight, gender, and height, is to get their RMR tested.

The process of checking your metabolism involves finding a place in your town that does resting metabolic rate testing, which estimates the number of calories burned at rest to determine baseline caloric needs. It also provides a measure of fat and carbohydrate utilization.

Specifically, the test involves breathing into a tube for ten minutes or so while a machine measures the amount of oxygen you are consuming. The more accurate tests require you fast twelve hours beforehand, and are typically not cheap, starting at $70. They also are not covered by insurance companies, so you have to come out of pocket if you really want to verify a fast metabolism – something most people are not pressed to do.

As I said before, some people do have higher metabolisms than others. The biggest influencer on our metabolic rate is our body size. This enables men to have higher metabolism across the board because they are normally bigger, and have more lean muscle and larger organs than women. Women can thank our layer of subcutaneous fat, which is pretty hard to get rid of, for a lower metabolism since fat burns fewer calories than muscle.

Of course, we are not comparing you to men, we are talking about other women with the same stubborn layer of subcutaneous fat, smaller organs, shorter heights and fewer muscle. If you were to compare your metabolism to that of a woman of similar stature, age, weight, the difference would be insignificant. Find another woman of the same age and height, but markedly slimmer and she will have a lower metabolism. That, my friends, is the honest truth.

Naturally, some of you might be wondering about metabolic disorders such as hypothyroidism, or more fittingly, hyperthyroidism, which is caused by an overactive thyroid and causes substantial weight loss to those who suffer from this illness. According to experts, hyperthyroidism only causes about a three to four percent change in BMR. This means the average person suffering from this issue is only at a disadvantage of about 50kcals per day, or about one slice of bacon.

It is worth pointing out that there is a misconception that a fast metabolism equals a ticket to eat all the junk food known to man without the worry of gaining weight. This is not true. If you ever do find someone with a genuinely faster than average metabolism, a rarity, know that while they can eat more than most people without gaining weight, they can also gain weight if they over eat too.

The more likely scenario a person with a great body who you see chowing down on all the foods that got you into the predicament you are in is they eat very little the rest of the time you are not around, or they are utilizing what is known as NEAT. NEAT stands for non-exercise activity thermogenesis, and includes all activities that we would not consider exercise, but that make us vibrant independent beings.

Have you ever met a skinny person who just could not sit still? If so, then you have seen NEAT at work. Non-exercise activity varies by as much as 2,000 calories per day. While high-energy people are burning more calories, we are not talking about someone shaking their leg making that much of a difference.

Generally, occupations and leisure activities account for the difference, as some jobs are far more energy expending than others and leisure activities range from almost complete rest to non stop activity for those that are highly energized. Think about those who claim their hobby is watching Netflix versus those whose hobby is Frisbee. The calories burned doing these activities are the difference between night and day.

Sure enough, when the skinny people you see do over-feed, their changes in NEAT tend to account for the energetic counter response to fat gain by moving around more – at work, play, and fidgeting and moving around. Again, that is a marked difference from overweight people who might over feed and instead of moving more, go and take a nap. Nine times out of ten, this is really what is at play here, not some super lucky person with an abnormally naturally faster metabolism.

The main point you should takeaway from this chapter is that your metabolism is not a fixed entity that determines your weight regardless of how much eat or exercise. Neither is it something you cannot do anything about.

How fast or slow your metabolism operates is entirely based on the calories you burn, which you have tremendous control over. Therefore, you can stop cursing your fate, and start doing the exact same things the skinny women your height, weight, and age is truly doing to keep her figure.

Chapter 7 – A Little Assistance

Help - we all need a little of it sometimes, but many of us do not like to admit it. Whether it is from wanting to keep our trade secrets to ourselves or being ashamed that we were not able to accomplish something entirely alone, oftentimes the help we receive goes unacknowledged.

Honestly, I have never understood the shame in requiring or obtaining assistance. Most of my other books have been about detailing the many resources available to help you reach your goals easier and faster. Clearly though, everyone does not feel the same way. Hence, why so many thin women do not come forward about the help they have received that is partially responsible for their amazing physiques.

Obviously, some methods are more drastic and harmful than others. For example, you would be surprised at the amount of skinny girls walking around who have gone under the knife and owe their figures to the skill of a surgeon and his cannula. Other kinds of help come in the form of dieticians, personal chefs, private trainers, and meal prep services. Then there are other who abuse diet pills, drugs, alcohol, cigarettes, laxatives, saunas, and fasting to look the way they do.

Even when you do find someone willing to divulge some of the help they have had, you will never know the whole truth about all the different factors that have contributed to the final product you see before you at the moment. There is no one clear path to being skinny, and given the attitudes about dieting and slimming down, those who have carved out a path are not generally rewarded for it, so they keep mum.

You will get answers like, "I eat healthy," or "I keep active," but you generally will not hear, "I got cryolipolysis" or "I fast for two days out of the week," Yet the former are pretty popular amongst tons of svelte women. In fact, liposuction was number three in the top five surgical procedures performed in 2014 (210,552 procedures, up 5 percent from 2013).

As I touched on before, the majority of women possessing enviable bodies are dieting, counting calories and/ or watching what they eat. Their assistance comes in the form of diet programs like Atkins, Paleo, Intermittent fasting, Weight Watchers, IIFYM - better known as if it fits your macros, waist training garments that snatch their waist, and even Photoshop. Oftentimes they aim for under 1200 calories per day (the magical number touted in every article as the only way to avoid starvation).

When it comes to exercise, personal trainers are also a pretty big source of assistance in many a skinny girl's final results. They provide a huge source of motivation and accountability. There is a misconception that only celebrities and wealthy individuals can afford the luxuries of a personal trainer, but that simply is not true.

With the rise of live streaming over the Internet, many people are choosing virtual trainers over physical ones. This allows for an experienced and knowledgeable professional to watch you and correct you when you are wrong without having to pass on the cost of transportation and cost of living to you, as many virtual trainers can live thousands of miles away in a much cheaper city or town.

If you would prefer a real live trainer, no matter what your budget there's probably a way to afford one. Most trainers offer less expensive alternatives than individual private sessions. For example, some have semi-private sessions, where you and one or two other people share the cost, but still get a personalized plan.

Additionally, there is the option of hooking up with a trainer for five or ten sessions to get the layout for what they are prescribing, learn the proper way to perform exercises, etc. Then, when you are comfortable, you can take it, go off and make it your own. The direct feedback and having a program tailor made for you can truly make a world of difference in getting started on your journey.

When we get into more socially frowned upon assistance, like plastic surgery, there are many options and the decision of whether or not to explore those options is yours to make. After all, you are the only person who has to live in your body, so the choice to do or not do something to it should be entirely left up to you. I am of the opinion that if you want it, can afford it and understand that after the procedure you will need to do something different so as not to end up right back at square you, then go ahead.

Every year there are new breakthroughs in body contouring through surgical and non-surgical procedures. Machines, lasers and techniques are improved and/or developed, the costs become more reachable for the average working class person, and the results just get more and more impressive. We all know about liposuction, but there is also CoolSculpting, Vanquish, Sculpsure, transculpting, lipolight, etc.

At the moment CoolSculpting, Vanquish, and Sculpsure are the most popular choices on the market, with the latter two being the more effective and less painful new kids on the block. There are pros and cons and similarities and differences amongst them that should be taken into consideration given your unique objective and current body.

CoolSculpting is older technology that destroys fat cells by freezing, which can result in bruising, numbness and unpleasant tingling sensations. Given its suction cup like application it can only be used to treat one area at a time and is ideal for localized areas of fat. Each area takes about an hour.

Vanquish destroys fat cells with heat, or more specifically, focused field radio frequency, without injuring other tissues or touching the patient's body. In contrast to Coolsulpting, Vanquish utilizes a large panel that lies very close to the skin and can cover a broad area or multiple areas at once. Treatment occurs in thirty to forty-five minutes. It can cause mild discomfort, but generally less pain overall versus Coolsculpting according to patients.

SculpSure uses an FDA-approved non-invasive laser device that leverages controlled and targeted hyperthermic laser. It is the only device in the world, as of this writing, that uses a laser (1060 mm) to permanently remove pockets of fat and can treat up to four areas in twenty-five minutes.

With this option, the lasers energy heats the fat cells and surrounding tissues. Patients feel warmth over the areas as with the Vanquish. Also like Vanquish, the treatment is incredibly effective and pain-free. There is no downtime and patients can return to work or other activities after treatment.

In all cases, the fat cells are destroyed, the body's lymphatic system carries away the cellular debris, and it is excreted. Multiple treatments are required before you will see results for Coolsculping and Vanquish. It reportedly takes one to three applications to get the full benefit of Coolsculpting, which each area taking an hour to treat, and four to six treatments for Vanquish. One session of Sculpsure will take six to twelve weeks to see the results.

All of these procedures have been proven to permanently destroy fat cells, although neither device removes as much fat as surgical liposuction. The main benefit though, is that these procedures are non-invasive, more cost effective, have less risk compared to liposuction, and are very effective at fat reduction, with a reported twenty percent to thirty percent destruction of fat cells.

If you are stumped about which procedure to get, Coolsculpting is best for more focused bothersome areas of excess fat, Vanquish is good for larger abdomens and it also has an application that specifically addresses fat reduction on the thighs, and Sculpsure is ideal for people looking to remove smaller pockets of fat. If you are pain averse and time pressed, Vanquish and Sculpsure are definitely the best option for you.

Now, if these options are not ideal for you because you have more than just small pockets of fat, or you have pockets of fat that do not change with diet and exercise, liposuction is probably your best option. There have been several surgical innovations, including laser-assisted liposuction (Smart Lipo, Cool Lip), water assisted liposuction (Body Jet), Power assisted liposuction, and ultrasonic assisted liposuction, that are supposed to make the removal of fat process less traumatic.

These procedures use cannulas that generate heat, vibration or ultrasound waves that break apart the fat cells before they are removed, but the fact that you are still receiving liposuction and still undergoing surgery still remains – and surgery should never be taken lightly.

The above are the only effective options outside of diet and exercise that exist that can help you lose fat today, and a lot of the women you see killing their spin class or carrying around yoga mats have utilized them, although they would never admit to it. Whether or not they decide to share the help they may have received, or keep it a secret does not really matter, or at least it should not matter to you.

For example, if an actress actually admitted that the real secret to her impressive weight loss was a bunch of cocaine and cigarettes, would you go and follow suit? Hopefully not, since you know that would be more harmful than helpful.

Sure, it would be nice if they gave credit to a fantastic doctor where it was due so you could go out and book an appointment. However, we have to deal with reality, and the reality is most people like to keep the measures they have gone to in the effort to improve their bodies under wraps. You can certainly choose to be vocal about your choice to enlist help, but you can also choose to keep your decision private and that might enable you to relate to your tight-lipped skinny sisters.

Chapter 8 – Hunger

"I forgot to eat today," "I'm craving a salad," "I'm still full from breakfast" or "I have a very small appetite". These are some of the more common reasons skinny women are known to give regarding the primal urge we all have to deal with when faced with trying to lose weight. I am talking about hunger, and their apparent lack of it.

Chances are you have pondered how someone could ever forget to eat a meal, much more multiple meals, over the course of an entire day. The idea is completely foreign and hard to relate to with the general public at large when there are restaurants, café's, coffee shops and bakeries on nearly every block, endless food commercials and advertisements on your social media feeds, television screen and streets, and apps that can have a hot meal delivered at your doorstop in less than fifteen minutes. Seriously food is everywhere and we are always being reminded of it, so forgetting about it for more than ten seconds might understandably seem insane.

Are these lies thin women have convinced themselves of, or use to get well and/or ill meaning friends who are trying to force food and alcohol on them, or are some thin people really perpetually full from very little amounts of food? If you chose the former, you would be correct!

First of all, it is only right to disclose upfront that there are certainly some instances where a person's appetite could wane that have nothing at all to do with his or her size. For example, we all know for a fact that some people react to anxiety, stress or depression by pushing their plates away. This is generally because they feel a lack of motivation or energy that translates over to food. Additionally, there is the possibility that one's stomach might have a hard time accepting or processing food while he or she is extremely stressed, so food loses its appeal to some people going through a rough patch.

We can also add stomach bugs or the flu as possible explanations for a loss of appetite. Intuitively our bodies mount a complex inflammatory response to illness that involves producing chemicals called cytokines, which have a wide range of effects and are partly responsible for the decreased appetite.

When you are not chowing down and digesting, you free up energy to fight an infection or illness. Plus, if you find yourself with impaired smell and taste, as many people do when they get sick, a whole element of enticement is removed from the feasting experience.

Outside of these instances it is completely normal to feel hungry more than once a day as it takes six to eight hours for a meal to digest. Some of the factors that determine when you will be hungry include how much and how recently you last ate, social situations, the time of day, convenience, the times you typically eat, the smell and sight of food, and your emotional state. Of course, energy needs is a given, but for most of us the impetus to eat is rarely if ever based on the biological deficit or need such as insufficient glucose.

Slender women are every bit as human as the rest of us so they are not immune to the above. However, they do exercise a lot of self-control, have a different attitude about hunger, and employ tactics, deliberate and non-deliberate, that regulate their hunger a lot more effectively than heavier individuals. The good news is you can copy them to receive the same benefits.

There is a saying that goes, "An idle mind is the devil's playground". It means anyone with too much time on their hands may find themselves in hot, troubled waters or reaching for calorie dense, fat laden foods if we apply the quote to the context of this book.

It is hard to fathom being bored today with increasing workloads and deadlines, the Internet, apps, and gadgets we all seem to own that are designed to grab our attention and occupy hours of our time. If we are all busier, how come not all of us are forgetting to eat throughout the day? The answers are pretty obvious actually. First, despite all these distractions many people are more bored and unfulfilled than ever, so they look for satisfaction or comfort in food.

Those who keep themselves busy with work they are engrossed in are able to avoid the eat whenever bored trap so many get caught in. I am not suggesting that all skinny people are perfect beings that do truly important work or that they are never idle. Of course they do, but the first step to removing food from the center of your universe is filling your world with important things – preferably that you really like to do or care about.

Now, even when you do find a way to preoccupy yourself that gets you into a nice flow from which you never want to leave, it is not unusual to expect to become hungry after a little while. It is not that your slimmer peers do not feel hunger or remember they have not eaten in a while, it is that they still prioritize getting whatever it is they are working on done over food, and most importantly, they know that hunger pangs come and go, buying them time.

That last sentence is the kicker and one I want to really sink in. Look, if you want to join the skinny crowd, you need to learn to embrace hunger instead of thinking of it as some state of emergency. Feeling hungry is healthy despite the notion in our society that it is a condition needs to be cured immediately. For one, hunger allows you to really enjoy your food. Second eating only when you are truly hungry helps to cut back on eating as much food. Third, you can still function just fine when you are hungry.

Before anyone gets up in arms, I should clarify that obviously hunger needs to be eradicated in places where food insecurity is a problem. However, hunger every now and then for people who are consistently in a state of overfeeding is not a bad thing in a place like America and other developed countries where there is plenty of food available to eat.

The problem is that most people munch all day long and never give the body time to become hungry. If you are like the majority of people who eat when not hungry (e.g. out of boredom, habit, or societal pressure), then you probably do not even know what it feels like to be hungry. The difference with a lot of thin people is that they typically do not eat unless they are truly hungry, and once they start eating they do not try to stamp out hunger forever by overeating to the point of combustion.

We now know that when a skinny woman says she forgot to eat for the day or was so busy she could not stop for food, that she is not being entirely truthful. Odds are, her body reminded her of its lack of food with a few well-placed tummy grumblings. Realistically, we know she could have fit a few minutes into her busy schedule to refuel if she really wanted to. The truth is hunger just does not rule every aspect of her life and actions, so they can continue working or playing and eat on their own terms.

You will not die the few hours between your meals when you give your mouth and tummy a rest. In fact, you will probably notice it only for a second before the feeling passes. If you choose not to dwell on the feeling or how to kill it, or obsess about the pang in any way, soon enough it passes.

You may find the idea of suppressing hunger odd or impossible. However, being thin is all about control, and although some people criticize this notion, confusing it with obsessiveness, it is far better than having no self-control. Taking control of your choices means you are serious about your goals, while being obsessive is control taken to the extreme - where your diet rules your thoughts, mood, and life.

Are there many skinny women who got that way from being obsessive (eating disorders and kicking themselves when they go off course)? Sure. Are there many skinny women who got that way through healthier measures such as setting goals for themselves and sticking to them while functioning in the rest of their life to the capacity? Absolutely!

To illustrate to those of you skeptics out there how hunger could be a good thing I would like us to look at intermittent fasting. With the rise of intermittent fasting over the years, we have come to learn more about the actual health benefits of being hungry every now and then. For example, in one recent study in Cell Metabolism, intermittent fasting was linked to lower risks of heart disease, diabetes, cancer and aging.

Besides the obvious fact that learning to embrace hunger ad eschew feeling full all the time aids in weight loss (you are eating less often and presumably consuming fewer calories), going without food improves insulin sensitivity and the immune system by reducing free radical damage.

It also improves your brain function by boosting the production of a protein called brain-derived neurotrophic factor (BDNF), which activates brain stem cells to convert into new neurons and protects the brain from changes associated with Alzheimer's and Parkinson's disease.

Finally, if you currently suffer from binge eating or excessive eating patterns, it is possible that you are not receiving the correct hormonal signals to let you know when you are actually full. Allowing yourself to finally experience true hunger can assist in resetting your body so that it can regulate itself to release the correct hormones and allow you to stop eating when you should. An added benefit to fixing this problem is that when your hormones finally start working properly, you will also find yourself getting full quicker.

It does take some adjusting to, especially if you have gotten used to frequent snacking (every two to three hours), and it will feel uncomfortable – more often at the start than ever, but it will get easier. There are so many diets that are dedicated to weight loss by avoiding hunger, but it is honestly more practical to embrace that hunger is a part of being skinny.

Of course, there are people who are starkly opposed to the idea of allowing yourself to ever get hungry. In their minds, when you're hungry your body is telling you to eat, so you must do so right away. Otherwise, if you let your hunger build up, you will fall down a binge-eating pit.

It is important to note that I am not advocating starvation, and there is a chasm of difference between hunger and starvation. Too many people think of hunger as not being full, so that when they actually are hungry (if they ever allow themselves to get there) they think they are starving.

Starvation occurs when a person cannot supply his or her body with adequate nutrition over a longer timeframe, usually weeks or months. It causes physical and mental side effects due to a prolonged lack of nutrition. Whereas hunger is the body's natural urge to replenish its food stores over the course of a day or two.

Hunger is not a villain, just a signal that your body is running low on its immediate supply of energy. It is worth mentioning though, that your body has a lot of reserve or back up energy in the form of body fat. However, half the time what people call hunger is actually the feeling of not being full, so their bodies actually have a lot of glucose to draw energy from and they can stand to go a few more hours without food.

I mentioned in the beginning of the chapter how oftentimes the people we think should be the hungriest based on their body fat use a lack of hunger is used as an excuse to get well or ill meaning friends from practically trying to force feed them. Whenever I am out in social situations and food is involved, which is nearly almost always, ladies who are thin will rarely eat the junk food almost always exclusively being offered.

I would like to stress that contrary to what skinny girls may tell you, it is not always easy to do what you set out to do. If you lose a little control – it is not the end of the world and it is nothing to get incredibly upset over. Acknowledge it and self correct the next day. A big secret skinny girls have is encouragement from online and offline communities reinforcing her to keep going. Most of the time we seek these friends or spaces online out.

For example, it is common for my thin friends and I to admit to eating a little bit too much the day before and thus alter our plans instead of eating out together. This is taking control of our actions and reinforcing each other's goals to keep our bodies light and tight.

I do not dismiss a friend's attempt to self correct by saying how silly she is being, and that eating again will not hurt her because she already has a great body. I know the reason for her shape is precisely because she has that awareness of what eating too much junk food will do to ones body and exercises moderation, and I am supportive of her decision. Unfortunately, this is something overweight and obese individuals have not mastered.

Therefore, refusing food – especially really tasty fried, cheesy, or sweet foods, around these individuals is a cause for investigation. To ward off the food police, it is just easier to say you are not hungry, just ate, or have a small appetite, even when it is not necessarily true, so you can stick to your diet plan without being rude or inviting people to offer their personal opinion on your diet.

Last, but not least, there are tactics that are known to regulate hunger. I discuss many of these tactics thoroughly in my books, *The Thigh Gap Hack* and *Bye-Bye Thunder Thighs*, and have even coined the phrase hunger training because it helps you reset and normalize your hunger cues.

While I cannot go into the entire protocol here, I can say that eating certain foods that are high in protein and fiber, moderate in fat, and low in sugar (including artificial sugar and sugar alcohols) and carbohydrates (grains), will allow you to stay fuller longer as you try to stretch out your meals. Specifically, the fiber helps you feel full right away, the protein helps you stay full for longer, and the fat works with your hormones to tell you stop eating.

Another part of hunger training involves scaling back on hyper palatable foods, a category all junk foods fall into. These are foods that taste so good because they are usually high in fat, sugar, and salt, or a combination of all three, which you crave more even when your tummy feels like it could burst from all the food you have eaten. It is why you can still find room for dessert even after a three course meal, or a whole bag of cookies is a breeze to tear through compared to a whole grilled chicken.

You would also be surprised at what your body craves and even enjoys once you give up foods that are awful for you for a month or more and then try to eat them again. Yummy cakes will suddenly taste sickeningly sweet and chips will taste so salty you might get a headache. In other words, the magic appeal does wear off once you get your taste buds to come back down to earth.

My last tip for surviving hunger is to create obstacles between yourself and easy access to food. Let's face the facts; you are more inclined to eat when food is literally right at your fingertips than when not. One Cornell researcher found proof that the out of sight, out of mind and mouth temptation factor exists in a study where women were found to eat more than twice as many Hershey Kisses when they were in clear containers on their desks than when they wee in opaque containers on their desk – but fewer when they were sex feet away.

Some real world ways to apply what we learned from this study, and my favorite, is to leave the house without any money. No cash, credit cards, gift cards – nothing. By doing so, I am guaranteed to avoid making purchases on the whim. I also only visit the grocery store twice a month instead of weekly, which cuts down on having to resist buying tempting foods by half.

If you work for yourself, it might mean cancelling delivery service sites like Seamless or Grubhub so it is not as easy to order out, having no junk food in the house, and preparing your meals and snacks for the day from the night before. If you like to work remotely, it might mean ditching the coffee shops where you are tempted to get pastries for a jolt of energy every few hours and going to libraries, parks, or bookstores instead or only bringing enough cash to buy a cup of coffee.

If you really love sweets, creating obstacles might be as simple as making a deal with yourself that you will only eat sweets that you bake yourself, and/or only making enough for one serving. Finally, a really relevant one in this day and age – unlike and unfollow all food accounts on social media and block or avoid watching food centric television channels.

These are just a few ideas to get you started on how to make food less accessible or off your subconscious and conscious mind. With some thought I am confident you can think of more solutions that are targeted to your situation and specific weaknesses.

Chapter 9 – Meal Frequency

The recommendation for how frequently you should eat is ever changing. A while back we were all being told to eat three square meals a day, then it changed to five or six meals a day so as to supposedly increase metabolic rate, then intermittent fasting entered the ring and eating one or two meals a day became the in thing.

The rub is that during every phase there have been skinny people who swear by one plan over the other, which should tell us that it actually has no bearing on being slim. Therefore, anyone who uses meal frequency as the reason for her admirable body did not get that way because she eats six tiny meals, or because she has a five-hour eating window. There is nothing magical about either.

If you are still not convinced, let's look at one of the prevalent ideas that says you have to eat breakfast if you want to avoid entering the world of plus sized clothing. Well, in order for that to be true you simply have to disprove it once. If you eat breakfast and still struggle with your weight, that is one big clue eating or skipping breakfast is not the be all end all of weight management.

Beyond that, although there have been many observational studies showing statistical links between breakfast skipping and obesity, a 2014 randomized controlled trial that involved 238 overweight and obese adults, found there was no different in weight between groups who ate breakfast versus those who skipped breakfast over sixteen weeks.

Next, is the six small meals a day mantra, which was originally popular amongst the bodybuilding community as a way to massive gains before being turned into weight loss advice. What fueled its popularity is the idea that every time you eat, the body burns calories to digest the food (thermic effect of food or TEF for short), so eating meals more often should increase metabolic rate and allow the body to burn more calories overall.

TEF means the body expends a certain amount of energy digesting the nutrients in a meal, and amounts to about twenty to thirty percent of calories for protein, five to ten percent of calories for carbs, and zero to three percent of calories for fat.

However, we have since learned it doesn't quite work that way. While it is true that TEF is a real thing and on average you can burn ten percent of your total calorie intake because of it, whether you eat six two hundred calorie meals or two six hundred calorie meals, you will still get a thermic effect of ten percent, or one hundred and twenty calories in both cases. It is the total amount of calories consumed, not how many meals you eat that make the difference.

Yet another reason someone might advocate eating more frequently is that it will keep hunger at bay. Besides the fact that we already talked about hunger not being this villain you need to stave off at every moment, the evidence from several studies that have actually looked into this claim is hardly conclusive.

Some suggest more frequent meals lead to reduced hunger, others find no effects, and still others show increased hunger levels – so that only thing that is certain is that eating frequently to reduce hunger depends on the individual.

The only reason you should eat a bunch of little tiny meals per day is if you find that it reduces your hunger over the course of the day. I suspect the quality of the foods you are eating is what would have the most effect on that though. If meal number one is cake, and meal number two is popcorn, you can bet your hunger will not be headed in the trajectory you want it to.

Now, just because eating a lot does not appear to be the saving grace some think it is, doesn't mean skipping meals is the obvious way to turn either. Unfortunately, as fasting or intermittent has caught on with the general public, people have just flipped the script to painting the method itself as the answer instead of one of many means to an end.

For example, eating one meal a day is still certainly not quite mainstream, but you might find some people who have adopted this eating pattern because they are convinced it will undoubtedly keep them in great form. I can promise you that if you are eating once but consuming calorie dense foods such as ice cream or pasta with five cheeses that amount to more calories than you burn, you will not lose a single pound.

Furthermore, intermittent fasting or doing one meal a day is again not the cure all for everyone as some people report experiencing issues such as binging or overeating, low energy, headaches, and other undesirable side effects while others thrive without a single issue at all. There may also be psychological difficulties that arise from such infrequent feeding that may lead some people to the point of obsessing about food and when they can eat next.

Even my favorite way of eating, intermittent fasting where you eat however many times you want in a window of time up to a certain amount of calories, is not the golden ticket to being skinny. Sure, it helps me control the amount of calories I take in by preventing me from snacking at night when most people are susceptible to overeating, but it may not work for someone with a different lifestyle (e.g. job, workout plan, sleeping pattern, and family responsibilities).

My suggestion is that you take a look at your eating pattern at the moment and try something different for a few weeks to a month. After all, if your current eating style has not been working for you all this time, you have nothing to lose.

So if you are a six small meal a day person but you are still struggling with your weight, you might try three larger meals; if you are a one meal a day person, maybe divide up your feast into two meals over the course of the day. Yes, you can even give five or six small meals a whirl to see if that suits you better.

Most importantly, make sure you track your calorie consumption, food choices, and body metrics while you are testing out your new meal plan. There will not be drastic changes in your weight or measurements in the couple of weeks, but you can note and compare how full or hungry you feel, whether you make healthier or unhealthier choices when you switch your meal frequency, and whether the plan simply fits with your unique lifestyle.

There is no right or wrong way, just the best way that works to keep your overall calories low. For some, eating often prevents hunger cravings and binging on high calorie and/or junk foods. Others consume fewer calories by eating three square meals a day because they spend less time thinking about and preparing meals and more time on hobbies, work, etc.

Remember, meal frequency is only important when the context of what the person is eating at each meal is considered and how they react to the protocol. We must realize the complexities of human metabolism and patterns of different types of people play a huge role in weight loss and management.

Chapter 10 - Health

I could have ended the book with the last chapter, but I thought it would be irresponsible to ignore the big elephant in the room, which is health. Being healthy means truly taking care of oneself and not just looking externally healthful.

The assumption is that skinny equals healthy and that thin people are healthier. Logically, we know leanness is not the sole marker of health, yet the idea is perpetuated by the fact that most thin women who are suffering from health issues that directly result or contribute to their leanness, tend to keep this information under wraps.

It seems pretty straightforward why people might want to lie about their health. They do not want to focus on what is wrong with them, and it is a depressing issue. Most people would also prefer not to broadcast their health issues or struggles because they consider it a weakness and are trying to protect their self-esteem or prevent word from spreading. On top of this, for many people ignorance is bliss so not only are they lying to those around them, they are in fact lying to themselves about their problems.

You can be skinny and unhealthy because you only eat junk food (yet still burn more calories than you ingest) but your body is not getting the nutrients it needs to function optimally. You can be thin and beautiful but be skinny fat and have a high risk of disease like high cholesterol, diabetes, and arterial plaque.

You can look amazing in designer sample size clothes but suffer from disorders such as excessive exercising, weight obsessions, anorexia, bulimia, orthorexia (an obsession with eating foods that one considers healthy), and other forms of disordered eating.

You can be the perfect weight and height with lots of followers and likes on social media but deal with depression, extreme food sensitivities or allergies (e.g. celiac disease), illnesses such as cancer or immunodeficiency diseases, and addictions to drugs and cigarettes.

Everyone could envy your figure but when you look in the mirror you may see a distorted version of yourself – one that needs to lose more weight, fix this or that, because you have body dysmorphic disorder.

I think we can all agree that despite all the above examples having a gorgeous body in common, they are far from healthy or leading healthful lives. Again, we all know this, but yet we still have a tendency to look at skinny women and wish we could be like them because we perceive their lives to be easier and better – and oftentimes their public persona confirms and contributes to this picture.

Now, sometimes the truth gets brought to light about the very unhealthy issues skinny people may be facing. This is very common in the entertainment industry. A rising star or a star at the top of her game with a stunning body will deny and defend herself against whisperings of an eating disorder or drug problem only to fess up to being miserable and starving herself at the time years later. We have seen this with Nicole Ritchie, Lindsey Lohan, Nicole Scherzinger, and there are just too many more to mention.

You might admire how these people look but you have no idea of the suffering a person may be enduring. When you ask them to reveal the secret to their amazing physique, you will get a generic or canned response like the many we have covered so far instead of a candid reply.

Health is one of the most important things in our lives. Unfortunately, most people will not realize the importance of their health or fully appreciate their health until it is compromised. Poor health will both reduce the time you have in this world and your capability to live the live you want to.

Although it might look like all skinny women are leading amazing, glamorous lives, you simply do not know exactly what is going on behind closed doors. I say all of that to stress the importance of losing weight the right way instead of resorting to shortcuts that you think will expedite you to greener grass.

There is nothing wrong with admiring other women's bodies or having image boards displaying your goal body – better known as Pinterest. Images of yourself at a lower weight and others that inspire you are proven to increase motivation and help carry you towards your goals. For example, you might be more inclined to decline donuts after checking out a few snaps of your favorite fitness personality or super model.

Where many go wrong is when they beat themselves up for not getting to the same weight of a celebrity fast enough. Sometimes people who have been working hard and seeing results, still get frustrated when they do not look exactly like they thought they would. Remember, you will never be privy to all the details of how or why someone has been able to achieve a certain look.

Besides the fact that I hate the idea of unattainable bodies - we hear this word being thrown about a lot when it comes to getting skinny, because I know for a fact that everyone has the ability be slender, you still have to be realistic about certain things.

For example, if you are a shorty like me, you will never have super long legs like Giselle no matter how much weight you lose. And while some people are naturally able to be super lean and still have full boobs, the majority of us will lose the fat in our breasts the leaner we get. This means if you are trying to look like Pamela Anderson in her heyday, you are probably going to need implants because beasts are made up of fatty tissues, and when we lose fat it goes from the desirable and undesirable places alike – unless we are talking about getting help from a doctor.

It really all boils down to being patient - you did not put on the weight overnight and it will not come off overnight either, staying the course, and not compromising your health. I started this book out by telling you that skinny women value being thin, but while you want to prioritize it over a temporary sweet it is not to be valued over your health and life.

If you see yourself going down the wrong path, stop and reassess. Seek help from a professional if need be, but do whatever it takes to get out of the rabbit hole. You have a responsibility to take care of your body; it's the only one you will get in this lifetime and you truly cannot enjoy the perks of being thin if you are dying just to remain a certain size.

Chapter 11 – Welcome to the Other Side

Congratulations, you have made it to the end of the book, or what I like to call the other side because now that you know these hidden truths there is no going back to the dark. I hope I have been able to answer your questions and remove the shroud of mystery that surrounds the slim and trim, while clearing up a lot of misconceptions floating around about what it actually takes to join the ranks of this group of women.

I also hope now that I have spilled the T or tea (code word for truth), as they say, and you are armed with the knowledge of how skinny women really think, act, and communicate, what they eat and do not eat, and how that may differ from what you do, you realize whatever weight or size you are striving to be is completely possible. No good genes or lucky super charged metabolism necessary, just knowledge and the will to change your habits.

Wrapping it All Up

The last thing I want to point out is that while it may seem unnecessary, weird, or wrong for some people to lie about the things we have covered in the book, and even worse for them to lie to someone who is asking so that they can try to replicate the results, you have to realize that it is not done with malicious intent. What you are seeing is simply self protection and preservation at its finest.

If you recall I mentioned at the beginning of this book the women whose bodies you admire are not forthcoming for what they perceive to be valid reasons. Some may actually believe the lies they are telling you because it is reinforced in popular culture, but the majority have ascertained that their honesty is not welcomed. As a result, outsiders are kept out of the loop. This means people who thin shame, encourage being overweight or obese because it's what a so-called real woman is, and thinks being thin and maintaining such a body is unrealistic or unattractive.

However, thin women's guards usually come down for anyone who they perceive to be like-minded and non-judgmental. In other words, people who are in their tribe - other skinny women, or those who are in the process of losing weight who do not police other's methods or buy into the conventional advice and handwringing about weight loss. I say all of this to say that if you want the skinny to stop lying and open up to you about their regimen, beliefs and mindset, you cannot be seen as the enemy or outsider.

On that note, you cannot phone it in either. Fakeness can be detected from a mile away. If you secretly begrudge or judge the very people you are asking for help or harbor feelings of jealousy or spite because they have the body you want, it will show. Therefore it is uber important that you get rid of any negative or ulterior attitude pronto.

Only then should you go about seeking and befriending the thin – and to be clear, you absolutely should do so. The saying, you are who you hang out with could not be any more true. It explains why you see squads of itty biddy women hanging out together, and squads of overweight women hanging out together. The company you keep reinforces your behavior big time.

If your crew never wants to workout or do anything active, or only wants to get together to experience the latest unhealthy food craze taking over social media (grossly sweet calorie bombs topped off with two or three whole desserts being passed off as milkshakes, anyone?), even if you resist a few times eventually you will start to give in. Peer pressure is real and mindsets are indeed contagious.

Vice versa when you go out with slender people and observe how they eat, you will be much more inclined to follow suit. Of course, if they are of the group that pigs out socially because that will be their only meal for the day, or they order a ton of food and take three-quarters of it to go (or leave it behind on the table), you can be aware of these behaviors that normally go unnoticed.

Other places where you can look for like-minded skinny girlfriends are in your fitness classes or gym. If you are a bigger person I understand it may be tempting to seek out someone whom you can relate to, but I repeat this is not the way to go. Find friends that are already successful in the area you are seeking to change and you will be happy you did. Once it is obvious you are a skinny girl waiting to get out, you will be embraced.

Now, if you are having trouble finding real life skinny friends to associate with, there are some things you can do. First, whenever you go out, try to eat near someone who is thin and observe her from afar. Second, turn to the world wide web. There are plenty of weight loss support groups out there. That being said, not all weight loss support groups are created equal. For those groups that do not vet their members, you are bound to find people who will scare off others from being candid and open.

Therefore, it is best to join a private group, preferably of women who have already slimmed down and are trying to maintain their weight or have just a few pounds left. This is where you will find practical advice and encouragement, compared to groups full of people just beginning their journey who do not know the things that you now know.

Pass the Baton

That being said, I have one simple favor to ask of you as you start your journey to skinny or when you finally get to your goal weight. Now that you know are on the other side with information that is normally kept close to the chest, please do not keep your newfound revelation to yourself.

There are other people out there, many whom you love and care for and are in the same boat as you, who stand to benefit from learning the truth.

You can bet hard your bottom dollar they will be hard pressed to hear any of these things we have just spent ten chapters covering directly from a thin woman, so the best thing you could do is share this information and enlighten them.

As a matter of fact, buy them this book as a birthday, Christmas or non-holiday related gift. This way not only will you be positively impacting the lives of people you care about, you can kill two birds with one stone and stop the incessant stream of well meaning but bad advice from friends or family who try to convince you that you should embrace your body the way it is or that it was meant to be a certain way.

If your friends and family will not listen to you and do not want to be enlightened, you can still help others who are actually receptive to changing for the better by simply leaving a review of this book on amazon.com, itunes.com, barnesandnobles.com or goodreads.com.

Your experience and opinion may be just what someone else on the fence needs to give this book a chance. That is all that is needed for the word to spread. Yes, your single review can literally help change the misleading beliefs about what it takes to be skinny and shape a new lifestyle for someone else all by taking a minute or two to share your honest opinion with other potential readers.

Lastly, as with all of my books, if you have any unresolved questions about going oil free or want clarification on any of the information contained within this book, feel free to reach out to me. My personal email is camille@thighgaphack.com. I am happy to help or just hear the success stories I am sure you will have to share.

For those of you who have more in depth questions or feel like you need help beyond the scope of this book, I have taught thousands of people how to lose weight (fat, unwanted overdeveloped muscle, and water weight for special occasions), and I can help you too. Again, you can email me directly to inquire about my consultant rates.

You may also want to check out my other books, *"The Thigh Gap Hack"*, my magnum opus that reveals some of the fitness industry's biggest and best kept secret shortcuts for slimming the biggest problem area for most women, *"Bye-Bye Thunder Thighs"*, which cover how to slim the thighs with a tight focus on diet, *"How to Lose Water Weight"*, a book I wrote that focuses more on quick weight loss techniques when you want to look good fast for a special occasion, and *"The Easy Diet"* (also known as The Oil Free Diet), which deals with how simply removing oil from your diet is one of the easiest actions you can take to lose weight as well as details how to transition to cooking and preparing foods without oil seamlessly.

Finally, as I have said time and time again, I love researching, talking, and writing about fitness and always have my fingers on the pulse of new happenings.

I usually share my latest findings, research, success stories, tools, resources, and favorite tips and tricks on fitness related topics - from fashion, food, gadgets and beyond, on my general newsletter, which you can sign up for at http://www.thighgaphack.com. You can also find me on

Facebook www.facebook.com/thighgaphack

Twitter www.twitter.com/thighgaphack

Instagram www.instagram.com/thighgaphack

and YouTube www.youtube.com/thighgaphack.

I look forward to connecting with you on any and all of these outlets.

###

Prelude to 'The Skinny Girl Bible'

Have you ever read a book claiming to hold precious secrets and answers to a burning topic or question you are interested in, only to find common knowledge fare that's either outdated, not applicable to real life, or not nearly comprehensive enough?

I have, and it's downright insulting and infuriating! So, when I set out to write *'The Skinny Girl Bible'*, I wanted to make sure the content was so real, relevant, and encompassing that it would have no choice but to be called the downright authority on the non-obvious rules thin women live by.

With a name like The Skinny Girl Bible, I think it's evident that I won't be holding anything back. You won't find just ten or so actual nuggets (in other words a listacle padded enough to be disguised as a book) here.

What you will find is over 100 fresh *commandments* (hard and fast rules like in the real bible) expounded upon so you not only get to see the way many thin women think, but plan, act and react to certain scenarios that result in them easily keeping the weight off. From page one, I jump straight to the point and there is so much to cover, you can rest assured that there is zero room for filler.

I chose this name for the book not only because it reflects a lack of brevity. The bible is the book of life, full of wise teachings, lessons and tenets that if followed will allow people to find happiness, peace and meaning in this world.

'The Skinny Girl Bible' has a similar objective: It is full of wise teachings and lessons from those who have successfully acquired what you want – confidence and happiness in their skin, and control over food that holds so many others captive, and gives you the step-by-step breakdown of how you can get it for yourself.